CELL SURFACE FACTORS, IMMUNE DEFICIENCIES, TWIN STUDIES

BIRTH DEFECTS: ORIGINAL ARTICLE SERIES

Daniel Bergsma, *Series Editor*

Volumes in the series published by Alan R. Liss, Inc.

1975 – VOLUME XI

No. 7 **Morphogenesis and Malformation of Face and Brain,** Jan Langman, *Editor*

1976 – VOLUME XII

No. 1 **Cancer and Genetics,** R. Neil Schimke, Robert L. Summitt, and David J. Harris, *Editors*

No. 3 **The Eye and Inborn Errors of Metabolism,** Anthony J. Bron and Edward Cotlier, *Editors*

No. 4 **Developmental Disabilities: Psychologic and Social Implications,** Ann E. Pulver, *Editor*

No. 5 **Cytogenetics, Environment and Malformation Syndromes,** R. Neil Schimke, *Editor*

No. 6 **Growth Problems and Clinical Advances,** R. Neil Schimke, *Editor*

No. 8 **Iron Metabolism and Thalassemia,** Anthony Cerami, Charles M. Peterson, and Joseph H. Graziano, *Editors*

1977 – VOLUME XIII

No. 1 **Morphogenesis and Malformation of the Limb,** Widukind Lenz, *Editor*

No. 2 **Morphogenesis and Malformation of the Genital System,** Richard J. Blandau, *Editor*

No. 3 **Annual Review of Birth Defects, 1976,** R. Brian Lowry, *Editor*
Proceedings of the 1976 Vancouver Birth Defects Conference.
Published in 4 volumes:

- 3A Numerical Taxonomy of Birth Defects *and* Polygenic Disorders
- 3B New Syndromes
- 3C Natural History of Specific Birth Defects
- 3D Embryology and Pathogenesis *and* Prenatal Diagnosis

No. 5 **Urinary System Malformations in Children,** John W. Duckett, *Editor*

No. 6 **Trends and Teaching in Clinical Genetics,** Frederick Hecht, Gerald H. Prescott, and Joan H. Marks, *Editors*

1978 – VOLUME XIV

No. 1 **Genetic Effects on Aging,** David E. Harrison, *Editor*

No. 2 **The Molecular Basis of Cell-Cell Interaction,** Richard A. Lerner, *Editor*

No. 3 **The Genetics of Hand Malformations,** by Samia Temtamy and Victor A. McKusick

No. 5 **Neurochemical and Immunologic Components in Schizophrenia,** Allan L. Goldstein, *Editor*

No. 6 **Annual Review of Birth Defects, 1977,** Robert L. Summitt, *Editor*
Proceedings of the 1977 Memphis Birth Defects Conference.
Published in 3 volumes:

- 6A Cell Surface Factors, Immune Deficiencies, Twin Studies
- 6B Recent Advances *and* New Syndromes
- 6C Sex Differentiation *and* Chromosomal Abnormalities

No. 7 **Morphogenesis and Malformation of the Cardiovascular System,** Glenn C. Rosenquist, *Editor*

IN PRESS

Sex Chromosome Anomalies in Children, Arthur Robinson, *Editor*

Recent Advances in the Developmental Biology of Central Nervous System Malformations, Ntinos C. Myrianthopoulos, *Editor*

The National Foundation–March of Dimes
Birth Defects: Original Article Series, Volume XIV, Number 6A, 1978

CELL SURFACE FACTORS, IMMUNE DEFICIENCIES, TWIN STUDIES

Part A of
Annual Review of Birth Defects, 1977

Sponsored by The National Foundation–March of Dimes at
The Hyatt-Regency Memphis Hotel
Memphis, Tennessee

Editors:

Robert L. Summitt, MD, Professor of Pediatrics, Anatomy and Child Development, University of Tennessee, Memphis

Daniel Bergsma, MD, Series Editor
The National Foundation

Associate Editors:

Park S. Gerald, MD, Department of Pediatrics, Children's Hospital Medical Center, Boston, Massachusetts

Alexander R. Lawton, MD, Department of Pediatrics, University of Birmingham, Alabama

Robert E. Tipton, MD, Assistant Professor of Pediatrics, University of Tennessee, Memphis

Natalie W. Paul
The National Foundation

ALAN R. LISS, INC., NEW YORK

To enhance medical communication in the birth defects field, the National Foundation publishes the *Birth Defects Atlas and Compendium,* an *Original Article Series, Syndrome Identification,* a *Reprint Series,* and provides a series of films and related brochures.

Further information can be obtained from:

The National Foundation
1275 Mamaroneck Avenue
White Plains, New York 10605

Published by:

Alan R. Liss, Inc.
150 Fifth Avenue
New York, New York 10011

Views expressed in articles published are the authors', and are not to be attributed to The National Foundation or its editors unless expressly so stated.

Library of Congress Cataloging in Publication Data

Main entry under title:

Cell surface factors, immune deficiencies, twin studies
(Birth defects original article series; v. 14, no. 6A)
(Part A of Annual review of birth defects, 1977)
Includes bibliographical references and index.
1. Immunological deficiency syndromes--Congresses.
2. Immunologic diseases in children--Congresses.
3. Diseases in twins--Congresses. I.Summitt, Robert L.
II. Bergsma, Daniel. III. National Foundation. IV. Series.
V. Series: Annual review of birth defects; 1977, pt. A.
RG626.B63 vol. 14, no. 6A [RC585] 616'.043'08s
ISBN 0-8451-1020-9 [616.07'9] 78-17058

Printed in the United States of America

THE NATIONAL FOUNDATION is dedicated to the long-range goal of preventing birth defects. Our interim goal is to search for ways to ameliorate those birth defects which cannot be prevented.

As part of our efforts to achieve these goals, we sponsor, or participate in, a variety of scientific meetings and symposia where all questions relating to birth defects are freely discussed. Through our professional educational program we speed the dissemination of information by publishing the proceedings of these meetings and symposia. From time to time, we also reprint pertinent journal articles to help achieve our goal. Now and then, in the course of these articles or discussions, individual viewpoints may be expressed which go beyond the purely scientific and into controversial matters. It should be noted, therefore, that personal viewpoints about such matters will not be censored but this does not constitute an endorsement of them by The National Foundation.

Contents

Contributors

Arthur S. Aylsworth [117]
Department of Pediatrics and Child Development Institute
University of North Carolina School of Medicine
Chapel Hill, NC 27514

Kurt Benirschke [179]
Department of Pathology
University of California, San Diego
La Jolla, CA 92093

Kare Berg [193]
Institute of Medical Genetics
Oslo, Norway

Colin M. Bloor [179]
Department of Pathology
University of California, San Diego
La Jolla, CA 92093

Baruch S. Blumberg [91]
The Institute for Cancer Research
The Fox Chase Cancer Center
7701 Burholme Avenue
Philadelphia, PA 19111

G. A. Bruns [1]
Department of Pediatrics
The Children's Hospital Medical Center
300 Longwood Avenue
Boston, MA 02115

Chung-Ho Chang [137]
Department of Pediatrics
Children's Hospital of Michigan
3901 Beaubien
Detroit, MI 48201

Harold Chen [137]
Department of Pediatrics
Louisiana State University School of Medicine
Shreveport, LA 71130

Joe C. Christian [167]
Associate Professor of Medical Genetics
Department of Medical Genetics
Indiana University School of Medicine
1100 West Michigan Street
Indianapolis, IN 46202

Peter Coccia [85]
University of Minnesota
Minneapolis, MN 55455

Max D. Cooper [49]
Department of Pediatrics
University of Alabama in Birmingham
University Station
Birmingham, AL 35294

The number in brackets following each contributor's name is the opening page number of that author's paper.

Linda A. Corey [193]
Department of Human Genetics
Medical College of Virginia
Richmond, VA 23298

Nuhad Dinno [213]
Associate Professor
Department of Pediatrics
University of Louisville, School of Medicine
Louisville, KY 40202

Jean S. Drew [91]
The Institute for Cancer Research
The Fox Chase Cancer Center
7701 Burholme Avenue
Philadelphia, PA 19111

Milton T. Edgerton [223]
Chairman
Department of Plastic Surgery
University of Virginia Medical Center
Charlottesville, VA 22901

V. Faber [131]
Department for Infectious Diseases M
State University Hospital of Copenhagen
Copenhagen, Denmark

James D. Folds [117]
Clinical Immunology Laboratory
University of North Carolina School of Medicine
Chapel Hill, NC 27514

Kazimiera J. Gajl-Peczalska [85]
University of Minnesota
Minneapolis, MN 55455

Park S. Gerald [1]
The Children's Hospital Medical Center
300 Longwood Avenue
Boston, MA 02115

Randall M. Goldblum [73]
Departments of Pediatrics, Pharmacology and Human Biological Chemistry and Genetics
The University of Texas Medical Branch
Galveston, TX 77550

Andrew Hamon [213]
Senior Resident
Department of Obstetrics and Gynecology
University of Louisville, School of Medicine
Louisville, KY 40202

Zwi Hart [137]
Department of Pediatrics
Children's Hospital of Michigan
3901 Beaubien
Detroit, MI 48201

C. J. Hedeskov [131]
Biochemical Institute A
University of Copenhagen
Copenhagen, Denmark

William H. Hoffman [137]
Children's Hospital of Michigan
3901 Beaubien
Detroit, MI 48201

G. F. Johnson [223]
Children's Medical Center
Dayton, OH 45419

Joseph Kaplan [137]
Department of Pediatrics
Children's Hospital of Michigan
3901 Beaubien
Detroit, MI 48201

David H. Katz [59]
Department of Cellular and Developmental Immunology
Scripps Clinic and Research Foundation
La Jolla, CA 92037

John H. Kersey [85]
Department of Laboratory Medicine and Pathology
184M Jackson Hall
University of Minnesota
Minneapolis, MN 55455

Alexander R. Lawton [49]
Department of Pediatrics
University of Alabama in Birmingham
University Station
Birmingham, AL 35294

W. Thomas London [91]
The Institute for Cancer Research
The Fox Chase Cancer Center
7701 Burholme Avenue
Philadelphia, PA 19111

Edward D. Lustbader [91]
The Institute for Cancer Research
The Fox Chase Cancer Center
7701 Burholme Avenue
Philadelphia, PA 19111

J. L. Marsh [223]
Departments of Pediatrics and Plastic Surgery
University of Virginia School of Medicine
Charlottesville, VA 22901

W. Laurence Marsh [9]
Lindsley F. Kimball Research Institute of the New York Blood Center
310 East 67th Street
New York, NY 10021

Virginia V. Michels [201]
Kleberg Center for Human Genetics
Baylor College of Medicine
Texas Medical Center
Houston, TX 77030

Gordon C. Mills [73]
Departments of Pediatrics, Pharmacology and Human Biological Chemistry and Genetics
The University of Texas Medical Branch
Galveston, TX 77550

N. Morling [131]
Tissue-Typing Laboratory
State University Hospital of Copenhagen
Copenhagen, Denmark

Ntinos C. Myrianthopoulos [151]
National Institute of Neurological Diseases and Stroke
National Institutes of Health
Bethesda, MD 20014

Walter E. Nance [193]
Department of Human Genetics
Medical College of Virginia
Box 330, MCV Station
Richmond, VA 23298

J. Arly Nelson [73]
Departments of Pediatrics, Pharmacology, and Human Biological Chemistry and Genetics
The University of Texas Medical Branch
Galveston, TX 77550

Mark E. Nesbit [85]
University of Minnesota
Minneapolis, MN 55455

Guy S. Perry, III [85]
University of Minnesota
Minneapolis, MN 55455

P. Platz [131]
Tissue-Typing Laboratory
State University Hospital of Copenhagen
Copenhagen, Denmark

Vincent M. Riccardi [201]
Clinical Director
Kleberg Genetics Center
Baylor College of Medicine
Texas Medical Center
Houston, TX 77030

Meinhard Robinow [223]
Department of Pediatrics
University of Virginia Medical School
Charlottesville, VA 22901

L. P. Ryder [27, 131]
Tissue-Typing Laboratory of the Blood-Grouping Department
State University Hospital of Copenhagen
Copenhagen, Denmark

Hernan Sabio [223]
Department of Pediatrics
University of Virginia School of Medicine
Charlottesville, VA 22901

Frank C. Schmalstieg [73]
Departments of Pediatrics, Pharmacology, and Human Biological Chemistry and Genetics
The University of Texas Medical Branch
Galveston, TX 77550

Lawrence R. Shapiro [219]
Director, Cytogenetics Laboratory
Letchworth Village Developmental Center
Thiells, NY 10984
and
Consultant in Genetics
Westchester County Medical Center
Valhalla, NY 10595

M.H.K. Shokeir [103]
Division of Medical Genetics
University of Saskatchewan
Saskatoon, Saskatchewan,
S7N OW8 Canada

Martin J. Shulman [219]
Departments of Pediatrics and Pathology
New York Medical College
Valhalla, NY 10595

Beatrice D. Spector [85]
Research Specialist
Department of Laboratory Medicine and Pathology
University of Minnesota
Minneapolis, MN 55455

A. Svejgaard [27, 131]
Tissue-Typing Laboratory of the Blood-Grouping Department
State University Hospital of Copenhagen
Copenhagen, Denmark

William W. Temple [179]
Department of Pathology
University of California, San Diego
La Jolla, CA 92093

M. Thomsen [131]
Tissue-Typing Laboratory
State University Hospital of Copenhagen
Copenhagen, Denmark

S. Thyme [131]
Tissue-Typing Laboratory
State University Hospital of Copenhagen
Copenhagen, Denmark

N. H. Valerius [131]
Department for Infectious Diseases M
State University Hospital of Copenhagen
Copenhagen, Denmark

John K. Whisnant [117]
Department of Pediatrics
University of North Carolina School of Medicine
Chapel Hill, NC 27514

William G. Wilson [117]
Department of Pediatrics and Child Development Institute
University of North Carolina School of Medicine
Chapel Hill, NC 27514

Lionel Zemek [219]
Departments of Pediatrics and Pathology
New York Medical College
Valhalla, NY 10595

SECTION I: CELL SURFACE FACTORS, THEIR RELATIONSHIP TO DISEASE SUSCEPTIBILITY

Genetic Determinants of Viral Susceptibility*

Park S. Gerald and G. A. Bruns

Since molecules of significant size are unable to penetrate cell membranes passively, viruses cannot reasonably be expected to do so. It is becoming increasingly evident that the process whereby a virus enters a cell is often specific for the given virus. Recently, evidence has also been obtained that entry is dependent on the products of specific cellular genes. In the sense that these genes are required for viral invasion, they can be termed viral susceptibility genes. This review will describe what is presently known about such susceptibility genes.

The limited range of species susceptible to infection by certain viruses provides an initial suggestion that specific genes are involved. Since the picornaviruses are among the most limited in the range of species they attack, it is not surprising that they have provided much of the initial information. As their name indicates, the picornaviruses are very small (20–30 nm in diameter) and have RNA as their genetic material [1]. The picornaviruses important to man have been assigned to various subgroups according to the clinical features they produce (Table 1) [2]. Within each subgroup, the viruses are further categorized according to their reaction with specific antisera. These antibodies react with the proteins in the viral capsule and block the invasion of susceptible cells by the specific virus. The several serotypes within each subgroup are identified by number. The three serotypes of poliovirus, for example, are designated types 1, 2, and 3.

The earliest studies leading to information on the genetic basis of cellular susceptibility to viruses were performed with poliovirus. These studies were greatly aided by the ability of cultured cells from man and certain primates to support the multiplication of poliovirus in vitro [3]. This permitted examination of the range of susceptible species in the absence of organismal factors,

*This study was supported in part by NIH grants HD 04807, HL 10436 and HD 06276.

Birth Defects: Original Article Series, Volume XIV, Number 6A, pages 1–7

TABLE 1. Picornaviruses Infecting Man [2]

Classification	Number of serotypes
Enteroviruses	
Polioviruses	3
Echoviruses	31
Coxsackie viruses A	23
Coxsackie viruses B	6
Rhinoviruses	circa 100

such as the route of entry and the immune defense mechanisms. In this way the limited species range of susceptibility for poliovirus was found to be determined primarily by cellular factors [4]. Insusceptible cells from, say, the mouse, could support the multiplication of poliovirus, however, once the virus penetrated the cell membrane. This penetration could be induced by several means, such as by exposing the cells to naked viral RNA [5] or by trapping the virion within a lipid vesicle which is then taken up by the cell [6]. These findings demonstrated that the difference in susceptibility between various species is primarily the result of differences in the cell membrane.

The steps involved in penetrating the membrane of a susceptible cell are perhaps manyfold, but only two phases have been delineated so far. These are generally referred to as viral attachment and viral engulfment [2]. In many of the studies to be described, susceptibility of the cell to a virus has been judged by cell killing and/or viral multiplication. Both of the aforementioned phases of viral penetration of the cell membrane must therefore have occurred. For that reason, no attempt has been made in this review to equate the "susceptibility genes" with any individual membrane step.

Hybrid cells, derived from the combination of human cells with rodent cells (either mouse or Chinese hamster cells, both of which are insusceptible to many picornaviruses) have provided most of the critical information. Such hybrid cells are readily produced by fusing human cells (such as leukocytes) with an established rodent cell line. From these fused cells a hybrid cell will occasionally arise which contains the rodent genome essentially intact, but has only a few human chromosomes. These hybrid cells grow indefinitely in culture and may be examined both for their human chromosome content and for their susceptibility to viruses. When this was done, it was discovered that only those hybrids containing human chromosome 19 were susceptible to poliovirus [7–9]. No other human chromosome conferred susceptibility. Subsequently, it was shown that two other picornaviruses, Coxsackie B3 and Echo 11, likewise required the presence of chromosome 19 in order to invade the hybrid cell [10].

Current evidence suggests that there is a different susceptibility gene (or

TABLE 2. Effect of Isolated Erythrocyte "Receptor" on Enteroviruses [13]

Virus	Inhibition of: Infectivity (%)	Hemagglutination (titer)	Interpretation
Polio 1	0	–	Not inhibited
Echo 11	–	17	Not inhibited
Coxsackie B3	94	5,427	Inhibited

genes) on chromosome 19 for each of these viruses. This conclusion is derived principally from susceptibility studies of hybrids containing only a part of human chromosome 19. Hybrids have been produced, for example, from human cells obtained from a patient with the balanced translocation t(X;19)(q23 to 25; q13) (patient IX in Latt, Willard, and Gerald [11]). These hybrids were examined for their susceptibility to killing by various picornaviruses in the laboratory of Dr. John Enders (Ms. E. Grogan and Dr. J.F. Enders, unpublished data; Gerald, Monedjikova, and Enders [12]). Hybrid cells which contained only the 19pter to q13 portion of the chromosome were still susceptible to poliovirus (Types 1, 2, or 3). The susceptibility gene or genes for polioviruses are therefore located within this portion of chromosome 19. Similar experiments with Echo 11 virus, using these same hybrids, demonstrated that they were insusceptible to this virus. By inference, the susceptibility genes for Echo 11 are located in the 19q13 to qter region and are distinct from poliovirus susceptibility genes.

Similar tests of susceptibility to Coxsackie B3 virus were not carried out with these hybrids, but some information is available from published studies using isolated cell membrane fractions. Philipson et al [13] tested the ability of an erythrocytic membrane fraction to inhibit the hemagglutinating activity and/or the infectivity of polio 1, Echo 11 and Coxsackie B3 (Table 2). This particular membrane preparation was strongly inhibitory toward Coxsackie B3 but did not inhibit polio 1 or Echo 11. It is reasonable to conclude, therefore, that the susceptibility genes for Coxsackie B3 are different from those for polio 1 (and presumably also types 2 and 3) and Echo 11, even though the assignment of the Coxsackie B3 genes to a unique region of chromosome 19 has not been accomplished.

The finding that the first three picornaviruses studied in detail probably require independent susceptibility genes suggests that many different viral susceptibility genes exist. Further, the presence of these several susceptibility genes on the same chromosome might imply some common relationship among them, or with the other genes on this chromosome. The current gene map of this chromosome (Fig. 1), however, does not provide any support for this speculation.

The approach used for the study of picornavirus susceptibility is applicable

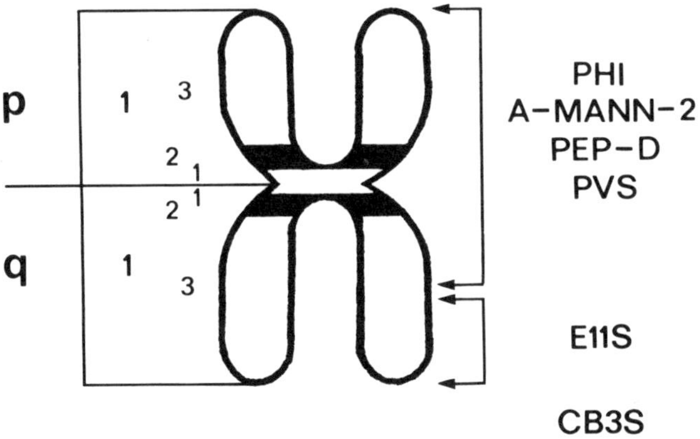

Fig. 1. Gene map of chromosome 19, summarizing presently available data from the authors' unpublished studies and from published reports [10, 31]. The loci indicated are poliovirus susceptibility (PVS), Echo 11 susceptibility (E11S), Coxsackie B3 susceptibility (CB3S), phosphohexose isomerase (PHI), lysosomal alpha mannosidase (A-MANN-2), and peptidase D (PEP-D). The regional localizations should be considered as tentative until independently confirmed. The regional location of CB3S is not known.

for the study of other viruses, when hybrids between susceptible and insusceptible species are available. From such studies, susceptibility to herpes simplex virus has been found to be dependent upon the presence of human chromosome 3 [14].

A different approach has provided information about influenza virus. The reaction of this virus with cells can be readily visualized because of its ability to agglutinate red cells. This hemagglutinating activity is inhibited in vitro by glycophorin, the major glycoprotein in red cell membranes [15, 16]. This suggests that influenza virus may bind to cells through its affinity for this membrane component. Since hybrid cell studies of susceptibility have not been done for influenza virus, there is no direct evidence for the number of susceptibility genes or for their chromosomal location. The chromosomal location of a gene, probably the structural gene, for human glycophorin is known, however, from the hybrid cell experiments of Puck and co-workers. They developed antibodies cytotoxic for cultured human cells by immunizing rabbits with human erythrocytes. One of these antibodies was found to react specifically with an antigen A_La_1, whose gene has been assigned to human chromosome 11 [17]. Most recently, this antigen has been identified with glycophorin [18]. If susceptibility to influenza

TABLE 3. Human Blood Group Loci Assigned to Specific Chromosomes

Blood group	Chromosome	Reference
Rhesus	1	21
Scianna	1	22
Dombrock	1	23
Duffy	1	24
Chido	6	25
Rodgers	6	26
Colton	7	27
Kidd	7	28
ABO	9	29
Enwright (glycophorin; $A_{L}a_{l}$)	11	18
Xg	X	30

virus proves to be dependent upon glycophorin and if susceptibility to this virus were to be examined in hybrids between human cells and cells of an insusceptible species, susceptibility should correlate with the presence of human chromosome 11.

Individuals who are Enwright blood group-negative are believed to lack glycophorin in their cell membranes [19]. If glycophorin is the only membrane component capable of attaching influenza virus to human cells, then Enwright-negative cells should be naturally insusceptible to this virus. Unfortunately, this possibility has not yet been subjected to experimental investigation.

The relation of the Enwright blood group system to glycophorin emphasizes the connection between blood groups and cell membrane components. Other blood group variants might, therefore, be associated with variation in susceptibility to certain organisms. As an example, erythrocytes that are Duffy blood group-negative are not invaded by certain malarial parasites [20]. Unfortunately, the current list of chromosomal assignments for blood group loci (Table 3) does not include any loci which are assigned to either chromosome 3 or 19, so that none of the alleles at these blood group loci would be expected to affect susceptibility to either polioviruses, Echo 11, Coxsackie B2, or herpes viruses.

As the preceding material demonstrates, evidence is available to support the view that genetic variation at loci for viral susceptibility genes can play a role in disease susceptibility. On the basis of current information, however, only a few individuals may have their susceptibility determined solely by such genes. On the other hand, the change in activity of susceptibility loci during development and differentiation may be influential in determining the clinical expression of viral diseases in the average individual. It is self-evident that inactivity at a susceptibility locus, as may occur normally because of the regulatory changes associated with differentiation or development, may result in a cell membrane lacking a component required for penetration by the infecting organism. Further study of this area may add much to our understanding of the clinical aspects of viral infection.

ACKNOWLEDGMENT

The authors are indebted to Dr. John F. Enders for advice and encouragement in these studies and in the preparation of this manuscript.

REFERENCES

1. Fenner F: Genetic aspects of viral diseases in animals. Prog Med Genet 8:1, 1972.
2. Fenner F, White DO: "Medical Virology." New York: Academic Press, 1970, p 265.
3. Enders JF, Weller TH, Robbins FC: Cultivation of Lansing strain of poliomyelitis virus in cultures of various human embryonic tissues. Science 109:85, 1949.
4. Holland JJ: Enterovirus entrance into specific host cells and subsequent alterations of cell protein and nucleic acid synthesis. Bacteriol Rev 28:3, 1964.
5. Holland JJ, McLaren LC, Syverton JT: The mammalian cell virus relationship. IV. Infection of naturally insusceptible cells with enterovirus ribonucleic acid. J Exp Med 110: 65, 1959.
6. Wilson T, Papahadjopoulos D, Taber R: Biological properties of poliovirus encapsulated in lipid vesicles: Antibody resistance and infectivity in virus-resistant cells. Proc Natl Acad Sci USA 74:3471, 1977.
7. Wang R, Pollack R, Kusano T, Green H: Human-mouse hybrid cell lines and susceptibility to poliovirus I. Conversion from polio sensitivity to polio resistance accompanying loss of human gene-dependent polio receptors. J Virol 5:677, 1970.
8. Medrano L, Green H: Picornavirus receptors and picornavirus multiplication in human-mouse hybrid cell lines. Virology 54:515, 1973.
9. Miller DA, Miller OJ, Dev VG, Hashmi S, Tantravahi R, Medrano L,Green H: Human chromosome 19 carries a poliovirus receptor gene. Cell 1:167, 1974.
10. Coullin P, Boue A, Rebourcet R, Van Cong N: Permissivite de clones cellulaires hybrides homme-souris a trois enterovirus: Poliovirus II, Coxsackie B3 et Echovirus 11. Pathol Biol (Paris) 24:195, 1976.
11. Latt SA, Willard HF, Gerald PS: BrdU-33258 Hoechst analysis of DNA replication in human lymphocytes with supernumerary or structurally abnormal X chromosomes. Chromosoma 57:135, 1976.
12. Gerald PA, Monedjikova V, Enders JF: Genes for susceptibility to viruses. Pediatr Res 8:424, 1974.
13. Philipson L, Bengtsson S, Brishammar S, Svennerholm L, Zetterquist O: Purification and chemical analysis of the erythrocyte receptor for hemagglutinating enteroviruses. Virology 22:580, 1964.
14. Garritt B, Goldfarb P: A human chromosomal determinant for susceptibility to herpes simplex virus. Nature 264:256, 1976.
15. Jackson RL, Segrest JP, Kahane I, Marchesi VT: Studies on the major sialoglycoprotein of the human red cell membrane. Isolation and characterization of tryptic glycopeptides. Biochemistry 12:3131, 1973.

16. Marchesi VT, Andrews EP: Glycoproteins: Isolation from cell membranes with lithium dilodosalicylate. Science 174:1247, 1971.
17. Wuthier P, Jones C, Puck TT: Surface antigens of mammalian cells as genetic markers. II. J Exp Med 138:229, 1973.
18. Moore EE, Jones C, Puck TT: Cell surface antigens IV. Immunological correspondence between glycophorin and the a_1 human cell surface antigen. Cytogenet Cell Genet 17: 89, 1976.
19. Dahr W, Uhlenbruck G, Leikola J, Wagstaff W, Landfried K: Studies on the membrane glycoprotein defect of En(a–) erythrocytes. I. Biochemical aspects. J Immunogenet 3: 329, 1976.
20. Miller LH, Mason SJ, Davorak JA, McGinniss MH, Rothman IK: Erythrocyte receptors for (Plasmodium knowlesi) malaria. Duffy blood group determinants. Science 189: 561, 1975.
21. Renwick JH: The Rhesus syntenic group in man. Nature 234:475, 1971.
22. Lewis M, Kalta H, Chown B: Genetic linkage between the human blood group loci Rh and Sc (Scianna). Am J Hum Genet 28:619, 1976.
23. Lewis M, Kalta H, Giblett ER, Anderson JB: Genetic linkage analysis of the Dombrock (Do) blood group locus. Winnipeg Conference (1977). Fourth International Workshop on Human Gene Mapping, Basel: S Karger for The National Foundation–March of Dimes BD:OAS XIV(4) In press.
24. Donahue RF, Bias WB, Renwick JH, McKusick VA: Probable assignment of the Duffy blood group locus to chromosome 1 in man. Proc Natl Acad Sci USA 61:949, 1968.
25. Middleton J, Crookston MC, Falk JA, Robson EB, Cook PJL, Batchelor JR, Bodmer J, Ferrara GB, Festenstein H, Harris R, Kissmeyer-Nielsen F, Lawler SD, Sachs JA, Wolf E: Linkage of Chido and HL-A. Tissue Antigens 4:366, 1974.
26. Gedde-Dahl T Jr, Robson EB: Rodgers blood group and the HLA region. Baltimore Conference (1975). Third International Workshop on Human Gene Mapping. Basel: S Karger for The National Foundation–March of Dimes. BD:OAS XII(7):311–312, 1976.
27. De la Chapelle A, Viropio P, Sanger R, Teesdale P: Monosomy-7 and the Colton blood groups. Lancet 2:817, 1975.
28. Shokeir MHK, Ying KL, Pabello P: Deletion of the long arm of chromosome No. 7: Tentative assignment of the Kidd (Jk) locus. Clin Genet 4:360, 1973.
29. Ruddle FH, Meera Khan P: Report of the committee on the genetic constitution of autosomes other than chromosomes 1, 2, and 6. Baltimore Conference, 1975. Third International Workshop on Human Gene Mapping. op cit, pp 31–53.
30. Mann JD, Cohan A, Gelb AG, Fisher N, Hamper J, Tippett P, Sanger R, Race RR: A sex-linked blood group. Lancet 1:8, 1962.
31. Ingram PH, Bruns GAP, Regina VM, Eisenman RE, Gerald PS: Expression of α-D-mannosidase in man-hamster somatic cell hybrids. Biochem Genet 15:455, 1977.

Chronic Granulomatous Disease, the McLeod Syndrome, and the Kell Blood Groups

W. Laurence Marsh, FIMLS, MIBiol

INTRODUCTION

X-linked chronic granulomatous disease (CGD) is caused by a defect in bactericidal function of the phagocytic leukocytes and is characterized by repeated, and sometimes overwhelming, infections. Some boys with X-linked CGD have red cells of the rare McLeod phenotype in the Kell blood group system. Red cells of this type show gross acanthocytic changes in morphology and have reduced in vivo survival. The McLeod phenotype is also inherited as an X-linked condition, and investigations have shown that the leukocyte anomalies of CGD, and the structural and blood grouping anomalies of the red cells that are associated with the McLeod type, arise from a common cause. In healthy individuals an X-linked gene called X^1k orders synthesis of an antigen called Kx on leukocytes and red cells. Antigen Kx is necessary for proper leukocyte bactericidal function and is a precursor structure utilized in production of Kell antigens on red cells. Inheritance of 1 of 3 variant alleles at the Xk locus (X^2k, X^3k, or X^4k) prevents synthesis of Kx either by leukocytes or by red cells, or by both, and is responsible for the cell structural and functional defects. The Xk locus is inactivated by Lyon effect, and female carriers of variant Xk alleles have a double population of functional and nonfunctional leukocytes, and of normal red cells of common Kell type and McLeod acanthocytes. The Xk locus is closely linked to the Xg blood group locus, and Xg^a red-cell typing in informative CGD families may provide valuable information for purposes of counseling.

Chronic granulomatous disease (CGD) is the name given to a disorder in which the main feature is high susceptibility to infection by low-grade bacterial

Birth Defects: Original Article Series, Volume XIV, Number 6A, Pages 9–25

pathogens [1]. The disease is characterized pathologically by sterile granulomata containing lipid-laden macrophages. A familial incidence of the disease was noted in early reports and the condition was believed to have an X-linked recessive mode of inheritance. Reports of female patients with CGD raised doubts concerning the genetic background of the condition [2], but it is now clear that at least one other defect may cause the same clinical syndrome. In the majority of cases the disease affects male children and is inherited as an X-linked condition from the carrier mother [3]. Affected boys show no evidence of any immunodeficiency disorder and have normal delayed hypersensitivity responses [2] and hypergammaglobulinemia [4]. The finding that immune mechanisms in these patients were normal prompted critical studies of the effectiveness of their phagocytic leukocyte function. Lysozyme and phagocytin enzymes of the leukocytes proved to be normal and the cells had normal phagocytic capability. The important finding was that although phagocytosis was normal certain intracellular metabolic changes which should accompany it did not occur [5], and the leukocytes had impaired killing power against several pathogenic and nonpathogenic organisms [6]. The clinical entity of X-linked CGD, in which a defect in bactericidal activity of monocytes and neutrophil leukocytes allows repeated, and sometimes overwhelming, infections thus became firmly established. Metabolic studies on leukocytes from these children show impairment in oxidative metabolism, in hexosemonophosphate shunt activation, and in generation of superoxide and hydrogen peroxide during phagocytosis. Phagocytosis by normal leukocytes is accompanied by a burst of cellular oxidative enzyme activity which is largely responsible for the cell's bacterial killing power [7]. Early studies on CGD leukocytes suggested that deficiency of oxidative enzymes might be responsible for the functional defect [8], but data from different investigations were somewhat contradictory. Studies on separated cell components have now confirmed the involvement of oxidative enzymes and have localized the abnormality to defective function of an NADH dehydrogenase present in the plasma membrane of neutrophil leukocytes [9]. The precise nature of the biochemical lesion that leads to the dysfunction, however, is still unknown. As with many inherited diseases, the severity in different individuals varies, although within a single family affected members show somewhat comparable degrees of disability. In the most severe form of CGD boys die from an infection in the first years of life.

CGD and the Kell Blood Groups

The Kell blood group of red cells was discovered by Coombs et al [10] in 1946. As with most blood groups, subsequent studies have revealed a complex system which at present includes about 20 different antigens (Table 1). The blood group is inherited in a straightforward manner as an autosomal dominant

TABLE 1. Antigens Related to the Kell Blood Group System*

Uncommon antigens	K	Kp^a	Js^a	K17	Ul^a				
Common antigens	k	Kp^b	Js^b	K11		K12	K13	K14	K18

*Kx is produced by an X-linked gene and is a precursor in the Kell biosynthetic pathway.

trait. A rare null phenotype, in which all Kell antigens are missing, was described by Chown et al [11] and named K_o. Family studies indicate that it arises by inheritance of silent K^o genes at the Kell locus from both parents. Another rare variant, in which the red cells show very weak antigenicity in the Kell system, was found by Allen et al [12] and named McLeod after the propositus. Family studies were at first uninformative in establishing the manner of inheritance of the McLeod phenotype.

Blood group notation is characterized by inconsistency and Allen and Rosenfield [13] proposed a numerical system for the Kell blood group in an attempt to create uniformity. The numerical terminology has been extended as new specificities have been recognized.

In 1969 a boy with CGD was reported to possess a red-cell variant phenotype in the Kell blood group system [14]. Other CGD cases involving variant Kell blood groups were described by Giblett et al [15] who pointed out that blood transfusions given to these children often provoked an antibody that reacted with virtually all random donor bloods. Early studies suggested that the Kell variant found may be either the K_o or the McLeod type, but differentiation between these 2 closely similar phenotypes is difficult to make without certain rare Kell system antisera. Recent investigations indicate that the variant seen is invariably that of the McLeod phenotype. Only 1 person in North America [12] and 2 in New Zealand (S. Shepherd and W.L. Marsh, unpublished observations, 1975) are known to have the McLeod phenotype without CGD and the findings in CGD cannot be due to coincidence.

One of the antibodies that helps differentiate these Kell phenotypes is anti-Ku [11]. This is found in the serum of immunized K_o people and is compatible only with other examples of the K_o type. The second informative antibody was found by van der Hart et al [16] in 1968, and named anti-KL. This antibody occurred in the serum of a boy whose red cells possessed weak antigens in the Kell system. He suffered from repeated infections and died subsequently from what, in retrospect, was probably chronic granulomatous disease. Red cells of common Kell types and K_o cells, which lack antigens of the Kell system, were all reactive with anti-KL, but McLeod-type red cells were compatible. The investigation by van der Hart et al [16] included antibody absorption studies using K_o red cells, with results which suggested that anti-KL serum may contain separable specific components. The observation that 2 antibodies might be present was confirmed by Marsh et al [17] who separated an example of anti-KL into two antibody fractions. The name anti-Kx (anti-K15 in numerical notation) was proposed for an antibody component that reacts strongly with K_0 red cells but extremely weakly with red cells of common Kell type. The second fraction, anti-KL, reacts strongly with red cells of common Kell type but is nonreactive with K_0 cells, a pattern of results which indicates that KL antigen is a product of the Kell gene. Anti-Kx makes a clear distinction between the McLeod and the K_0 red cell types, for McLeod cells lack Kx, while K_0 cells possess greatly increased amounts of the antigen.

Kx Antigen

The key to associating the Kell autosomal blood group system of the red cells with an X-linked defect of the phagocytic leukocytes proved to be anti-Kx. Marsh et al [17] were unable to detect the Kell antigens K, k, Kp^b, Js^b, K12, K13, or Ku on normal leukocytes, but demonstrated strong Kx activity using an antibody absorption technique. Tests on separated cell types from buffy-coat preparations showed Kx antigenicity with normal neutrophil leukocytes and monocytes [18], the 2 cell types that are functionally defective in CGD [6, 19]. Absorption of unprocessed anti-KL+Kx serum with normal leukocytes removed the anti-Kx component but left anti-KL, an experiment which confirmed the presence of Kx on leukocytes [17]. Investigation of defective leukocytes from CGD boys then established that they lack Kx antigen. Leukocytes from 50 normals were all Kx-positive, but 9 examples of X-linked CGD all had Kx-negative leukocytes [20]. The probability that this association would occur by chance is 7.95×10^{-11} (Fisher's exact method). The case for a direct association between lack of leukocyte Kx and the defect in bactericidal function is thus overwhelming. The 50 normal tests establish that the Kx-positive white cell phenotype has a minimum frequency of 0.94 (confidence level 95%), but it seems probable that the antigen is a fundamental property of normal phagocytic leukocytes. Although the biochemical nature of Kx is unknown, it appears probable that in leukocytes it is primarily involved in a trigger mechanism related to activation of NADH dehydrogenase in the cell membrane. Other leukocyte antigens are normal in CGD, and the abnormality relates specifically to the absence of Kx.

The Genetics of Kx

There is now ample evidence to show that Kx is produced by an X-linked gene. The observation that K_0 red cells have strong Kx allows the conclusion that the antigen cannot be produced by the Kell autosomal gene, for K_0 cells are homozygous for silent Kell alleles. The most reasonable explanation assigns Kx to the role of a precursor in the Kell biosynthetic pathway. Inheritance of silent Kell genes thus leaves a great excess of unconverted Kx as the only Kell-related antigen on the red-cell membrane.

Early studies to establish the manner of inheritance of the McLeod type were uninformative. But discovery of more examples in males, the absence of the phenotype in females, and the finding that the McLeod-producing locus is inactivated by Lyon effect, all indicate an X-borne mode of transmission. The weak Kell antigens of McLeod individuals differ qualitatively as well as quantitatively from the Kell antigens of other people [17, 21]. All of these findings indicate that lack of Kx precursor substance modifies expression of a normal Kell gene to produce the McLeod phenotype. Inheritance of the McLeod type thus reflects the genetics of Kx.

Frequency of the McLeod Phenotype

Tests on 6,150 random blood donors by van der Hart et al [16] using anti-KL+Kx serum did not reveal any examples of the McLeod type. If it is assumed that half of these were males it can be calculated that the KL-positive blood type has a minimum frequency of 0.9990 (confidence level 95%).

The McLeod type must be much rarer than this, however, for certain characteristic hematologic changes that accompany the phenotype would allow its recognition during routine laboratory examination of blood films. This aspect will be returned to later.

The Kell Biosynthetic Pathway

Race and Sanger [22] have proposed that more than 1 locus might be involved in production of Kell antigens and that the McLeod phenotype might result from a defect in a Kell precursor. Subsequent studies have confirmed this proposal of genetic complexity. The Kell phenotype of normal red cells arises by interaction between products of 2 independent genes (Fig. 1). One, named X^1k, is X-linked and controls synthesis of the precursor-like substance named Kx [17]. The Kell autosomal gene utilizes Kx substance in production of Kell antigens. The Kell gene itself may be a single regulated operon in which the antithetic pairs of antigens reflect different mutational sites in the structural region of the gene. While there is as yet no certain information to show which autosome carries the gene, the discovery that the Kell gene is closely linked to the gene *PTC*, which controls ability to taste dilute solutions of phenyl thiocarbamide [23], may be a start in assembling a Kell linkage group that may ultimately be informative in allowing assignment to a particular autosome.

Both normal leukocytes and normal red cells have been shown to possess Kx antigen. Red cells of common Kell type have only a small amount of residual Kx, which probably remains through incomplete conversion in the Kell pathway. Absence of the antigen in either cell type is a rare event. The finding in some

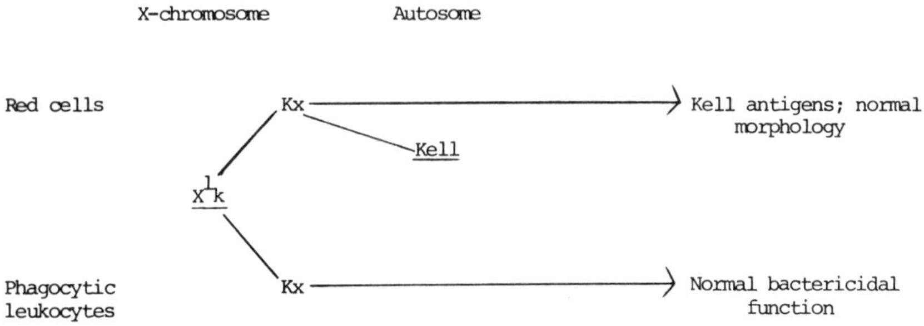

Fig. 1. A possible pathway of biosynthesis in the Kell blood group system.

boys that both cell types lack the antigen cannot be a result of coincidence and must be evidence that synthesis in both cell lines is ordered by the same structural gene. Most CGD boys with Kx-negative leukocytes, however, have Kx-positive red cells and common Kell phenotypes. Three males are known who have Kx-negative (McLeod) red cells but do not have the leukocyte dysfunction that causes CGD. Leukocytes from 1 of these have been examined and are Kx-positive [17]. In all of these cases family studies indicate an X-linked mode of inheritance. It appears, therefore, that the common allele called X^1k orders synthesis of Kx by phagocytic leukocytes and red cells in healthy people. Each of 3 rare variants, named X^2k, X^3k, and X^4k, at the same X-linked locus allows a different permutation of Kx synthesis in the 2 cell types [20]. Absence of leukocyte Kx is associated with a defect in bactericidal activity and CGD, while lack of red cell Kx results in the McLeod phenotype. These relationships are summarized in Table 2.

Hematologic Changes Associated With the McLeod Phenotype

Although blood group characteristics of the McLeod phenotype were recognized by Allen et al in 1961 [12], not until 1975 was it realized that the phenotype was associated with profound changes in red cell morphology and a hemolytic condition. Wimer et al [24] found that red cells from the first known McLeod person showed acanthocytosis and anisocytosis, and that the donor, although apparently healthy, had an enlarged spleen, reticulocytosis, reduced serum haptoglobin, and a compensated hemolytic state. The cell morphologic changes are readily discernible by light microscopy and are even more striking by electron microscopy (Figs. 2–4). Marsh et al [20] found the same acanthocytic changes in 5 other examples of the McLeod phenotype and Taswell et al [25] have reported a CGD boy with the McLeod phenotype, acanthocytic red cell morphology, and hemolytic anemia. The red cell anomalies arise by lack of Kx antigen and not through deficiency of Kell antigens. When viewed by either

TABLE 2. Phenotypic Effects That Result From Inheritance of Variant Xk Alleles

	Kx antigenicity		
Xk allele	Phagocytic leukocytes	Red blood cells	Clinical features
X^1k	Strong	Weak	Normal people of common Kell type[a]
X^2k	None	None	Type II CGD. Acanthocytic red cells with McLeod phenotype and shortened survival
X^3k	None	Weak	Type I CGD. Normal red cells of common Kell type
X^4k	Strong	None	Normal leukocyte function. Acanthocytic red cells with McLeod phenotype and shortened survival

[a] K_0 individuals have normal leukocyte Kx and an excess of Kx on their red cells.

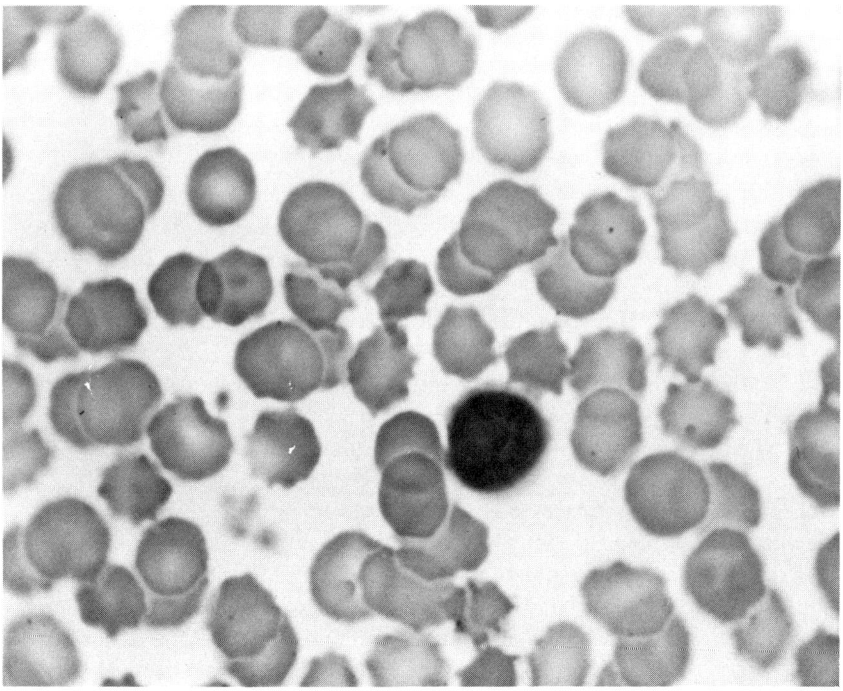

Fig. 2. Peripheral blood showing characteristic acanthocytosis of the McLeod syndrome (×1300).

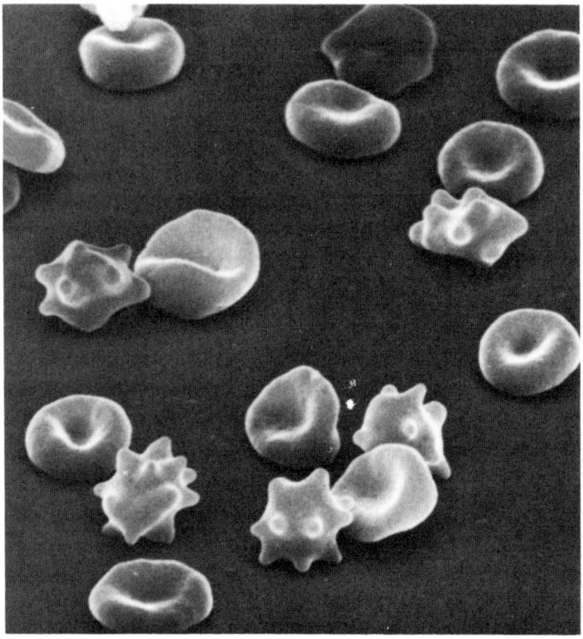

Fig. 3. McLeod syndrome red cells by scanning electron microscopy after immediate gluteraldehyde fixation.

light [20] or scanning electron [25] microscopy, K_0 red cells, which have strong Kx but lack Kell system antigens, are morphologically normal. Leukocytes from K_0 donors are also normal, both in their bactericidal function [15] and Kx antigenicity [17].

Other studies of McLeod-type red cells have established that although osmotic fragility is normal [24], the cells have decreased osmotic water permeability [26]. Individuals of McLeod type do not have abetalipoproteinemia, and their red cell lipid composition and cholesterol to phospholipid ratio are normal.

The i antigen strength of red cells increases during hyperactive red cell production [27]. Tests for i antigenicity on red cells from 2 CGD boys with McLeod phenotype by Marsh et al [20] showed enhanced activity, suggesting they had increased erythropoiesis. It was noted that CGD boys with McLeod-type red cells frequently required blood transfusions, but the need for transfusion was rare in boys whose red cells were of common Kell type. The previous clinical impression had been that the anemia in CGD was an effect of chronic sepsis, but it now seems probable that it results, in part at least, from abnormal survival of morphologically atypical red cells.

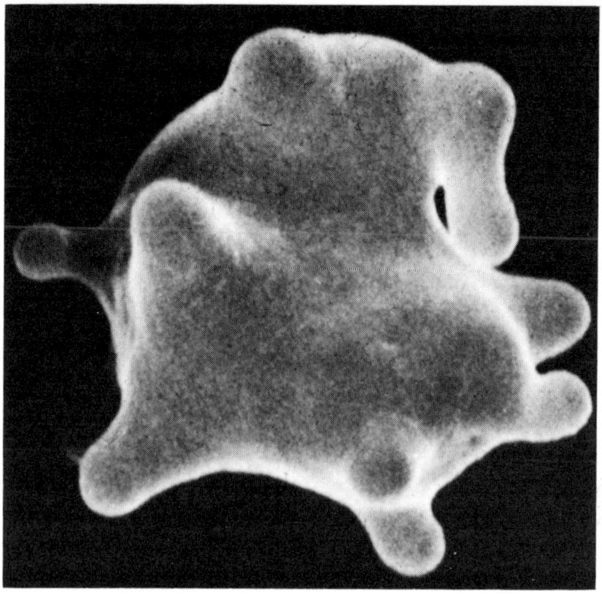

Fig. 4. A McLeod acanthocyte by scanning electron microscopy.

Type I and Type II CGD

Absence of leukocyte Kx antigen in X-linked CGD is not a secondary change caused by the disease, and the cell–membrane structure that carries the Kx antigenic marker appears to be one of profound biologic importance. Marsh et al [20] have divided X-linked CGD into 2 categories based on the presence of Kx antigen. Type I CGD has Kx deficiency which is restricted to the leukocytes, and red cell morphology in this case is normal. Type II CGD has Kx deficiency in both leukocytes and red cells, and as a consequence the granulomatous disease is accompanied by acanthocytic changes in red cell morphology and hemolytic anemia. The Xk variant genes responsible for these 2 clinical states are X^3k and X^2k, respectively. For those wishing to commit details to memory, it is convenient to remember that X^2k produces Type II CGD and is characterized by Kx deficiency in both cell lines. The great majority of CGD cases are of Type I.

Regulatory Changes Affecting the Kx-Producing Gene

In a general sense variant alleles at the Xk locus may be viewed as modifying genes of the Kell blood group system. The antigenic variation which results from hemizygous inheritance of a variant Xk allele must result from a regulatory change in the gene. Normal Kx synthesis in either leukocytes or red cells presumably requires the structural gene, and aberrant synthesis in either cell type must reflect a change in regulation. This effect cannot be caused by inheritance of an independently segregating modifying gene, for affected members of a single family always have the same pattern for Kx antigen synthesis. The variant allele must, therefore, be at the Xk locus. The human blood groups offer precedents for such inherited cell-specific modifications of structural gene activity. The A_m and B_m phenotypes in the ABO blood group, for example, are characterized by strong secretion of A or B blood group substances in saliva, which must require an A or B structural gene, but aberrant production of the antigen in red cells. Family studies establish that the phenotype may be inherited through an allele at the ABO locus [28]. In this situation, also, it must be assumed that the modified permutation of antigenicity between secretory tissues and red cells is caused by a tissue-specific change in gene regulation.

The McLeod Syndrome

Hemizygous inheritance of X^4k allows normal leukocyte Kx antigenicity but results in McLeod phenotype red cells with the associated clinical and hematologic complications. It seems appropriate to call these interrelated consequences of red cell Kx deficiency the McLeod syndrome (Table 3). Only 2 families are known in which some male members have McLeod syndrome without CGD. Shepherd and Marsh (unpublished observations, 1975) have studied a New Zealand family in which 2 males have McLeod syndrome with moderately severe hematologic effects, and 2 other male family members died from unexplained anemia at ages of 3 and 19 years. It appears possible that clinical manifestation of the McLeod syndrome may range from abnormal red cell morphology with a well-compensated hemolytic state to a severe hemolytic condition which may be fatal.

TABLE 3. Characteristics of the McLeod Syndrome

1) Red cells have the McLeod phenotype in which Kx is absent and Kell antigens are weak.
2) Red cells have acanthocytic morphology. Reticulocytes are increased and serum haptoglobin is reduced.
3) Clinical findings are an enlarged spleen and evidence of a hemolytic condition.
4) X-linked inheritance. The causative gene is carried by females and full expression is found only in males.
5) May be associated with leukocyte Kx deficiency and chronic granulomatous disease.

Xk Variant Alleles in Carrier Females

Windhorst et al [3] have reported that phagocytic leukocytes taken from mothers of boys with X-linked CGD comprise a double population of functional and nonfunctional cells. Marsh et al [18] found that carrier females have leukocytes with an intermediate level of Kx antigenicity, a finding that is consistent with a dual Kx-positive and Kx-negative cell population.

Swanson et al [29] demonstrated by quantitative studies that red cells from mothers of McLeod boys had weak k and Kp^b antigens. Marsh et al [30] subsequently found that these female carriers were blood group mosaics, having a mixture of common Kell and McLeod type red cells. The mosaicism is also detectable hematologically, for blood smears from carrier females show a mixture of normal discocytes and acanthocytes [24]. Figure 5 is a scanning electron microscope study of blood from a female carrier of the X^4k allele showing the double cell population. Careful blood group studies may be needed to recognize the mosaicism in female carriers who have relatively few McLeod red cells. In these cases the double cell population may be demonstrated more easily by identifying acanthocytes in a stained blood smear. In each of 7 female carriers of variant Xk alleles studied by W.L. Marsh, R. Øyen, and M.E. Nichols (unpublished observations, 1976), the population of red cells having common Kell type and normal morphology greatly outnumbered the abnormal cells that were

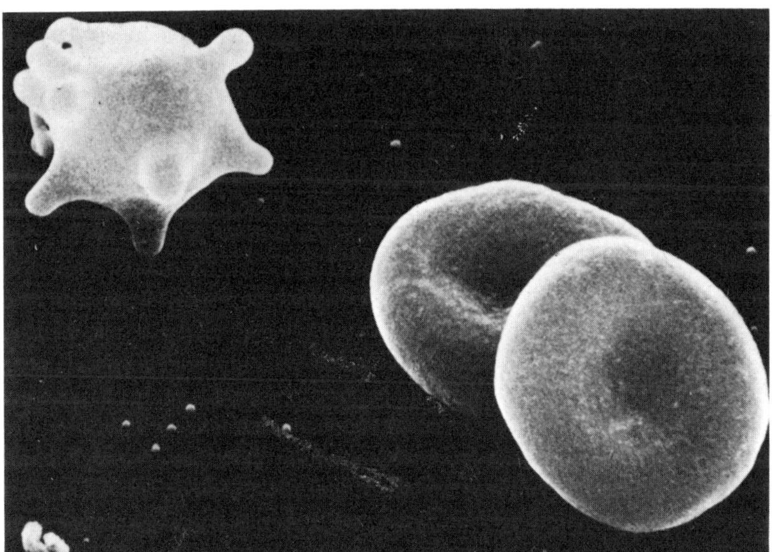

Fig. 5. Blood from an X^4k carrier female by scanning electron microscopy, showing normal red cells and an acanthocyte.

of McLeod type. The bias that favors normal red cells is unlikely to be a chance phenomenon and probably arises because normal cells have good survival in the peripheral circulation while the abnormal McLeod cells are prematurely eliminated.

Lyonization of the Xk Locus

Proof that the Lyon hypothesis [31] of X-chromosome inactivation applies to man was obtained by the demonstration that female carriers of variant glucose-6-phosphate dehydrogenase alleles are mosaics, having some cells with normal enzyme activity and a second population of deficient cells [32]. X-borne genes controlling some other enzymes have been found to follow the same pattern of expression.

The leukocyte and red cell mosaicism seen in females who are carriers of variant Xk alleles is attributed to the Lyon effect [3, 30], and the finding provides convincing support for assignment of the Xk locus to the X chromosome. The mosaicism also proves that Kx is a true red cell antigen and is not acquired by passive absorption from the plasma.

In man not all X-borne genes are inactivated by the Lyon effect. The X-linked Xg^a blood group provided significant information in this respect. It might have been expected that Xg^a *Xg* females would have a double population of Xg(a+) and Xg(a−) red cells. Because of technical difficulties, it took several years to establish that this was not so. Race [33], in 1971, concluded that females who are heterozygous at the Xg locus do not have a mixed Xg^a population of red cells and that the Xg locus is not inactivated by the Lyon effect. Wimer et al [24] and W.L. Marsh, R. Øyen, and M.E. Nichols (unpublished observations, 1976), have studied blood from Xg^a *Xg* female carriers of variant Xk alleles whose sons had the McLeod syndrome. All red cells in the double population present in the female blood were Xg(a+). Furthermore, when the normal red cells were removed by agglutination with anti-Kx serum, the remaining Kx-negative (McLeod) cells could still be typed as Xg(a+). It appears, therefore, that the Lyon effect on an X chromosome results in an inactive Xk locus but a functional Xg locus that can order production of Xg^a.

In 1975 Marsh [21] compared antigenic strength in the Kell system of red cells taken from normal males and females to determine whether the homozygous female produces more Kx and therefore has stronger Kell antigens. The study showed no significant difference between the sexes which is what would be expected in the light of the more recent discovery that one Xk locus in females is inactivated by the Lyon effect.

Linkage of the Xg and Xk Loci

Boys with CGD may be of either Xg^a type. Marsh et al [17] were unable to detect Xg^a on normal leukocytes using an antibody absorption technique. Although there is no evidence of any functional relationship between the products of the Xg and Xk genes, recent data have established that the 2 loci are closely linked. Race and Sanger [34] mention 2 Xg-nonrecombinant children in informative CGD families, which hints at possible linkage between the loci, and more nonrecombinants were added to the list through a CGD family study by Marsh et al [18]. Analysis of other informative families has now established the linkage ($\Theta = 0.00$ with a lod score of 3.426 [35]. (Lod scores are statistical methods, applied to data obtained from family studies, that indicate the likelihood of gene linkage. Scores greater than 3.0 give a high probability of linkage at the particular recombination fraction). Figure 6 shows the pedigree of a CGD family in which all affected sons are Xg(a+) and normal sons are Xg(a–). The variant X^3k gene in this family is traveling with Xg^a. If there is no linkage disequilibrium, about 45% of Xk carrier mothers will be heterozygous at the Xg locus, and therefore informative in using Xg^a to trace inheritance of the variant Xk gene. The fathers, of course, do not have to be considered in studies on boys suspected to have X-linked CGD. In those families where the father is Xg(a–) it will also be possible to use Xg^a typing to identify probable Xk variant carrier daughters.

The Relationship Between Kell and Kx

Little is known of the biochemical nature of antigenic determinants in the Kell system. Extraction of red cell membranes with n-butanol at 0°C leaves inhibitory activity for anti-k (and anti-K if the cells are K-positive) in the aqueous phase of the extraction. This suggests that some Kell activity is present as glycoprotein. But whether the carbohydrate or the protein moeity of the glycoprotein carries the specific determinant is not known. Discovery that a coliform organism which caused infantile enterocolitis produces a metabolite with Kell-like antigenicity allows some speculation. Infection with the organism stimulated production of apparent naturally occurring anti-K in the patient [36] Characterization of the bacterial K-like substance is in progress, but preliminary results indicate that it is polysaccharide in nature (W.L. Marsh, R. Øyen, and M.E. Nichols, unpublished observations, 1976). If the antigens of the Kell system result from immunodominant sugars, the Kell gene product must be transferase enzymes. The Kx antigen may, therefore, be a marker on a structural protein to which the Kell-specific sugars are attached. The limited information available concerning the biologic importance of blood group antigens indicates that loss of carbohydrate antigens does not alter red cell shape or survival [37, 38], but absence of an antigen such as Rh which is a marker of a membrane protein causes changes in red cell shape and decreased cell survival [38, 39]. The proposed Kell–Kx relationship is in accord with these general characteristics, and would explain why K_o cells, which may lack only Kell-specific sugars, have normal appearance and do not appear to have abnormal survival, while McLeod cells, which lack Kx, a possible structural protein, have changes in shape and reduced survival.

Non-X-linked Granulomatous Disease

On rare occasions, granulomatous disease affects girls [2]. In these cases blood group anomalies in the Kell system are not involved and the leukocytes do not lack Kx [20]. The disease in these cases is inherited as an autosomal recessive condition. A boy with this type of CGD studied by W.L Marsh, R. Clark, and S.J. Klebanoff (unpublished observations, 1976) had Kx-positive leukocytes. Although the clinical findings and leukocyte functional studies are similar, it appears probable that autosomal-recessive CGD is a different disease.

CONCLUSION

It is most unlikely that complex genes such as those of the blood groups would persist during evolution if their products did not play some advantageous

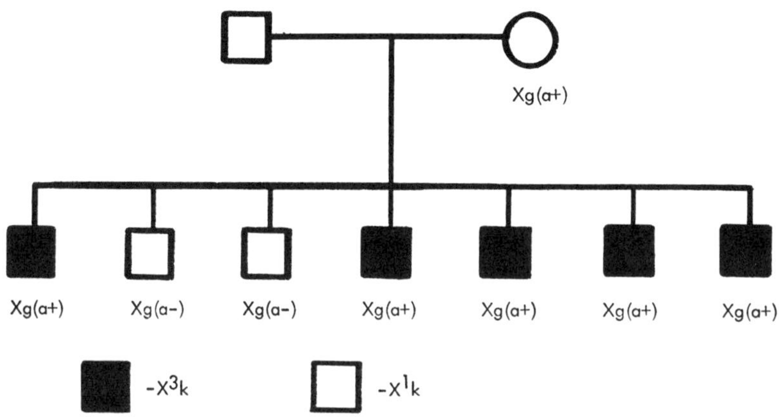

Fig. 6. Xg:Xk linkage. Part of an informative pedigree in which the X^3k allele is segregating with Xg^a. Male sibs only are shown.

functional role on the cell. Despite 70 years of blood group studies, only recently has it been possible to assign function to certain antigens. Absence of Rh antigens changes red cell shape [39], and the Duffy antigen has been identified as the membrane receptor used for invasion of the cell by the parasite of benign tertian malaria [40]. Although chronic granulomatous disease and the McLeod phenotype are rare conditions they are important, for their investigation has revealed that the Kx blood group antigen plays a vital functional role in red cells and leukocytes. Synthesis of Kx is ordered by an X-linked gene, and the fundamental defect in X-linked CGD must be failure to inherit X^1k. The enzymatic and functional disorders of the phagocytic leukocytes, and the structural changes in the red cells, are consequences which follow. Perhaps one of the most exciting facets of these investigations has been the discovery that the Xg and Xk loci are closely linked. The Xg^a antigen has been detected on red cells from fetuses aged less than 20 weeks [41], although the antigen increases greatly in strength later in fetal life [42]. For purposes of counseling, in about one-half of CGD families Xg^a red cell typing will allow recognition at birth of sons who have probably inherited the variant Xk gene. It is also possible that tests for Xg^a on fetal cells may allow the same recognition prior to birth.

The human blood groups have a wonderful complexity. The challenge to discover functional roles for other antigenic structures of the red cell lies before us.

ACKNOWLEDGMENTS

The cooperation of many clinicians and blood bankers who have referred CGD cases to our laboratory for investigation is gratefully acknowledged. I am also grateful to Dr. Bruce M. Wimer and to Dr. W. R. Galey who prepared the light and scanning electron microscope photographs of McLeod-type red cells.

REFERENCES

1. Bridges RA, Berendes H, Good RA: A fatal granulomatous disease of childhood. Am J Dis Child 97:387, 1959.
2. Azimi PH, Bodenbender JG, Hintz RL, Kontras SB: Chronic granulomatous disease in three female siblings. JAMA 206:2865, 1968.
3. Windhorst DB, Holmes B, Good RA: Newly defined X-linked trait in man with demonstration of the Lyon effect in carrier females. Lancet 1:737, 1967.
4. Janeway CA, Craig J, Davidson M, Downey W, Gitlan D: Hypergammaglobulinemia associated with severe recurrent and chronic nonspecific infection. Am J Dis Child 88: 388, 1954.
5. Holmes B, Quie PG, Windhorst DB, Good RA: Fatal granulomatous disease of childhood: An inborn abnormality of phagocytic function. Lancet 1:1225, 1966.

6. Quie PG, White JG, Holmes B, Good RA: In vitro bactericidal activity of human polymorphonuclear leukocytes: Diminished activity in chronic granulomatous disease of childhood. J Clin Invest 46:668, 1967.
7. Klebanoff SJ, Clem WH, Leubke RG: The peroxidase-thiocyanate-hydrogen peroxide anti-microbial system. Biochim Biophys Acta 117:63, 1966.
8. Baehner RL, Nathan DG: Leukocyte oxidase: Defective activity in chronic granulomatous disease. Science 155:835, 1967.
9. Segal AW, Peters TJ: Characterization of the enzyme defect in chronic granulomatous disease. Lancet 1:1363, 1976.
10. Coombs RRA, Mourant AE, Race RR: In vivo isosensitization of red cells in babies with haemolytic disease. Lancet 1:264, 1946.
11. Chown B, Lewis M, Kaita H: A "new" Kell blood group phenotype. Nature 180:711, 1957.
12. Allen FH, Krabbe SMR, Corcoran PA: A new phenotype (McLeod) in the Kell blood group system. Vox Sang 6:555, 1961.
13. Allen FH, Rosenfield RE: Notation for the Kell blood group system. Transfusion 1: 305, 1961.
14. Klebanoff SJ, White LR: Iodination defect in the leukocytes of a patient with chronic granulomatous disease of childhood. N Engl J Med 280:460, 1969.
15. Giblett ER, Klebanoff SJ, Pincus SH, Swanson J, Park BH, McCullough J: Kell phenotypes in chronic granulomatous disease: A potential transfusion hazard. Lancet 1:1235, 1971.
16. Hart MVD, Szaloky A, van Loghem JJ: A "new" antibody associated with the Kell blood group system. Vox Sang 15:456, 1968.
17. Marsh WL, Øyen R, Nichols ME, Allen FH: Chronic granulomatous disease and the Kell blood groups. Br J Haematol 29:247, 1975.
18. Marsh WL, Uretsky SC, Douglas SD: Antigens of the Kell blood group system on neutrophils and monocytes: Their relation to chronic granulomatous disease. J Pediatr 87:1117, 1975.
19. Davis WC, Huber H, Douglas SD, Fudenberg HH: A defect in circulating mononuclear phagocytes in chronic granulomatous disease of childhood. J Immunol 101:1093, 1968.
20. Marsh WL, Øyen R, Nichols ME: Kx antigen, the McLeod phenotype, and chronic granulomatous disease: Further studies. Vox Sang 31:356, 1976.
21. Marsh WL: Studies on the Kell blood group system. Med Lab Technol 32:1, 1975.
22. Race RR, Sanger R: "Blood Groups in Man." 6th Ed. Oxford: Balckwell Scientific Publications, 1975, p 302.
23. Conneally PM, Dumont-Driscoll M, Hartzinger RS, Nance WE, Jackson CE: Linkage relations of the loci for Kell and phenylthiocarbamide. Hum Hered 26:267, 1976.
24. Wimer BM, Marsh WL, Taswell HF, Galey WR: Haematological changes associated with the McLeod phenotype of the Kell blood group system. Br J Haematol 36:219, 1977.
25. Taswell HF, Lewis JC, Marsh WL, Wimer BM, Pineda AA, Brzica SM: Erythrocyte morphology in genetic defects of the Rh and Kell blood group systems. Mayo Clin Proc. 52:157, 1977.
26. Galey WR, Evan AP, Van Nice PS, Dail WG, Wimer B, Cooper RA: Morphology and physiology of the McLeod phenotype erythrocyte: I. Scanning electron microscopy and electrolyte and water transport properties. Blood (In press).
27. Hillman RS, Giblett ER: Red cell membrane alteration associated with marrow stress. J Clin Invest 44:1730, 1965.
28. Race RR, Sanger R: "Blood Groups in Man." 6th Ed. Oxford: Blackwell Scientific Publications, 1975, p 15.

29. Swanson J, Park B, McCullough J: Kell phenotypes in families of patients with X-linked chronic granulomatous disease. In "Abstracts XIII Congress, International Society for Blood Transfusion." Washington: American Association of Blood Banks, 1972, p 26.
30. Marsh WL, Taswell HF, Øyen R, Nichols ME, Vergera MS, Pineda AA: Kx antigen of the Kell system and its relationship to chronic granulomatous disease. Evidence that the Kx gene is X-linked. Transfusion 15:527, 1975.
31. Lyon MF: Genetic factors on the X chromosome. Lancet 2:434, 1961.
32. Davidson RG, Nitowsky HM, Childs B: Demonstration of two populations of cells in the human female heterozygous for glucose-6-phosphate dehydrogenase variants. Proc Natl Acad Sci USA 50:481, 1963.
33. Race RR: Is the Xg blood group locus subject to inactivation? In "Proceedings, 4th International Congress on Human Genetics." Amsterdam: Excerpta Medica, 1971, p 311.
34. Race RR, Sanger R: "Blood Groups in Man." 6th Ed. Oxford: Blackwell Scientific Publications, 1975, p 603.
35. Marsh WL, Allen FH, Øyen R, Mandel G, Kroovand S, Shepherd S: Linkage of the Xg and Xk blood group loci. (In preparation.)
36. Marsh WL, Nichols ME, Øyen R, Thayer R, Deere WL, Freed PJ, Schmelter SE: Naturally occurring anti-Kell stimulated by E. coli enterocolitis in a 20-day-old child. Transfusion (In press).
37. Seidl S, Spielman W, Martin H: Two siblings with Rh_{null} disease. Vox Sang 23:182, 1972.
38. Levine P, Tripodi D, Struck J, Zmijewski CM, Pollack W: Hemolytic anemia associated with Rh_{null} but not with Bombay blood. Vox Sang 24:417, 1973.
39. Sturgeon P: Hematologic observations on the anemia associated with blood type Rh_{null}. Blood 36:310, 1970.
40. Miller LH, Mason SJ, Clyde DF, McGinniss MH: The resistance factor to plasmodium vivax in blacks. N Engl J Med 295:302, 1976.
41. Toivanen P, Hirvonen T: Antigens Duffy, Kell, Kidd, Lutheran, and Xg^a on fetal red cells. Vox Sang 24:372, 1973.
42. Race RR, Sanger R: "Blood Groups in Man." 6th Ed. Oxford: Blackwell Scientific Publications, 1975, p 588.

The Role of the HLA System in Relation to Disease in Man*

A. Svejgaard, MD, PhD and L.P. Ryder, BS

Landsteiner's discovery of the ABO blood group system in 1901 [1] was the first step towards safe blood transfusion therapy in man, and it formed the necessary basis for many of the triumphs celebrated by today's modern surgery. A considerable number of other red blood group systems, most notably the Rhesus system [2], were found later which have further increased the safety of blood transfusion. While blood grouping serology has thus proved to be indispensable in practical clinical medicine and a powerful tool in human population genetics, it is a striking fact that very little is known about the biologic function of most of the red blood group systems although a picture is beginning to emerge for some [3]. In contrast, the first (*A*) *h*uman *l*eukocyte (HLA) system discovered by Dausset in 1958 [4] appears to control several vital immune functions [5, 6], and thus its existence is profoundly important. Although we are now probably seeing only the top of the iceberg, and although the HLA system has been recognized as one genetic system for only a decade [7], more is known about its biologic function than that of any human red blood group system. Accordingly, it is perhaps not surprising that the HLA system seems to play a much broader role in disease susceptibility than other genetic systems.

In this report, a brief review of the various components of the HLA system will be given. This will be followed by a more detailed discussion of the relationships which exist between this system and susceptibility to a variety of diseases. The role of the HLA system in clinical transplantation and blood transfusion will be but briefly mentioned since it has been dealt with recently in detail by others [8].

*This study was aided by grants from the Danish Medical Research Council, the Danish Blood Donor Foundation, and the Nordic Insulin Foundation.

Birth Defects: Original Article Series, Volume XIV, Number 6A, pages 27–46

THE HLA SYSTEM

Several recent reviews of the HLA system exist [9–12] and here we shall only summarize the most important points.

The property of the HLA system which led to its discovery was its ability to induce, after blood transfusion or during pregnancy, the formation of specific alloantibodies reacting specifically with alloantigens present on the leukocytes and platelets of the blood donor or the child. The reaction between antibody and and antigen has a number of consequences, one of which is the activation of complement which damages the cell membrane. This effect is the basis for the so-called lymphocytotoxicity test [13], the most common method for HLA typing. Microliter amounts of a lymphocyte suspension separated from a peripheral blood sample are mixed and incubated with sera containing known HLA antibodies, complement is added, and the reaction is read under the microscope after the addition of supravital stains (eg eosin or trypan blue), which enter cells with membrane damage.

An impressive number of HLA antigens has been discovered in this way (Fig. 1 and Table 1). They occur in a population with various frequencies and belong to three different segregant series named *HLA-A, -B,* and *-C.* All antigens are inherited as co-dominant characters and within each series behave as if controlled by allelic genes corresponding to three closely linked loci on the short arm of chromosome number 6 [14, 15]. The HLA-A, -B, and -C antigens each consist of two polypeptide chains [9]: one glycosylated with a molecular weight of

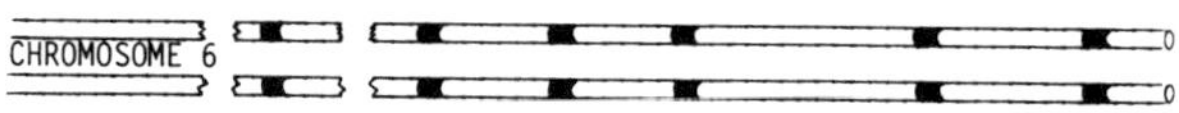

Locus: ←centromere	PGM_3	HLA-D	Bf	HLA-B	HLA-C	HLA-A
No. alleles:	3	>8	3	>20	>5	>17
Determinants:		HLA-Dw1		HLA-B5	HLA-Cw1	HLA-A1
		-Dw2		-B7	-Cw2	-A2
		-Dw3		-B8	-Cw3	-A3
		-Dw4		-B12	-Cw4	-Aw23 } A9
		-Dw5		-B13	-Cw5	-Aw24 } A9
		-Dw6		-B14	-T7	-Aw25 } A10
		-LD107		-B18		-Aw26 } A10
		-LD108		-B27		-A11
				-Bw15		-A28
				-Bw17		-A29 } Aw19
				-Bw21		-Aw30 } Aw19
				-Bw22		-Aw31 } Aw19
				-Bw35		-Aw32 } Aw19
				-Bw37		-Aw33 } Aw19
				-Bw38 } Bw16		-Aw34
				-Bw39 } Bw16		-Aw36
				-Bw40		-Aw43
				-Bw41		
				-Bw42		

Fig. 1. The HLA complex. The human major histocompatibility complex located on the short arm of chromosome 6. Genes for GLO, C2, and C4, and for the blood group Bg, Chido, and Rogers are also linked to HLA.

TABLE 1. Linkage Disequilibrium (gametic association)*

Haplotype			Frequency, %	
A	B	D	Observed	Expected[a]
A1	*B8*		9.8	2.1
A3	*B7*		5.4	2.1
	B8	*D3*	8.6	1.4
	B7	D2	3.9	1.8

*Data from Svejgaard et al [31].
[a]Calculated under the assumption of no association.

43,000, carrying the HLA antigenic determinant, and thus encoded for by an HLA gene on chromosome 6, and another which is beta-2-microglobulin (molecular weight = 12,000), the gene for which is on chromosome 15 [9].

In addition to the *HLA-A*, *-B* and *-C* antigens, the HLA system controls at least one other series of antigens, the *HLA-D* antigens. These differ from the former in several ways: While the ABC antigens are present on all cell types except red cells, the D antigens are primarily present on B lymphocytes, monocytes, endothelial cells, and sperm. The HLA-D antigens are also called MLC (or LD = lymphocyte-defined) antigens because they are responsible for the stimulation seen in mixed leukocyte cultures. The ABC antigens induced little or no detectable response in such cultures. The HLA-D antigens are probably identical or closely related to some of the so-called Ia (immune region-associated) or B lymphocyte antigens, which can be detected serologically in B lymphocyte-enriched suspensions [16, 17]. The Ia antigens also consist of two polypeptide chains with molecular weights of 33,000 (containing the polymorphic antigens) and 28,000 [9]. They are called Ia antigens because the corresponding antigens in mice [11] are controlled by genes mapping close to the so-called Ir (immune response) genes within the H-2 system (the mouse homolog of HLA). Each vertebrate species investigated has been found to possess its particular HLA analog. These systems control the immune response (more precisely IgG antibody production and cell-mediated immunity) to a variety of antigens [6]. The HLA system has not yet formally been shown to contain Ir determinants, but this is mainly due to the fact that planned immunization of humans with synthetic antigens is generally not considered ethical. However, the analogy between the HLA system and the corresponding systems in other species is so close that the HLA system almost certainly contains Ir determinants. This assumption is supported by circumstantial evidence, particularly the associations between HLA and certain diseases, to be discussed below. Moreover, it seems increasingly likely that at least some Ir, Ia, and HLA-D determinants may be identical (see below).

Finally, the HLA system has been found to control some components of the complement cascade. For example, the structural genes for the properdin-factor Bf, the second (C2), and the fourth (C4) complement components are closely linked to the HLA system [22].

When discussing HLA in relation to disease susceptibility, it is necessary to consider the phenomenon called linkage disequilibrium (illustrated in Table 1). An HLA haplotype is the set of linked HLA genes that has been inherited from one parent and which accordingly is located on one of a pair of chromosomes passed on to a descendant after meiosis. It is apparent from Table 1 that the *HLA-A1* and *B8* genes are present in the same haplotype about five times as often as would be expected if linkage equilibrium existed between the *A* and *B* loci. In analogy, *HLA-B8* and *Dw3* are also positively associated. In fact, these gametic associations exist for all HLA loci described so far, and they are reflected at the population level by associations between the corresponding antigens: eg individuals who are B8 are much more likely to be A1- and Dw3-positive than are B8-negative individuals. Accordingly, if Dw3 occurs with increased frequency in a group of patients with a particular disease, then A1 and B8 are also increased, and occasionally it can be difficult to decide which of the antigens shows the strongest association. Bodmer [9, 19] has recently surveyed the various explanations for the existence of linkage disequilibrium, and he favors the possibility that it is created by natural selection, on the assumption that certain gene constellations confer an advantage for the individual.

Biologic Function of HLA Factors

Obviously, the complement factors encoded by genes within the HLA system – like other complement factors – are important as part of the body's defense mechanisms against infection. However, not until recently has some light been thrown on the biologic role of the HLA antigens per se. Most of the accumulated knowledge has been obtained from animal studies, and there is increasing evidence that similar mechanisms operate in man. The discovery of H-2-linked Ir genes in mice [6] was a very significant step towards understanding the role of these systems. The function of *HLA-A*, *-B*, and *-C* antigens still remained in the dark until the exciting demonstration by Doherty and Zinkernagel [5] that the ABC equivalents of mice (the H2-D and -K) antigens serve a role by being part of the molecules on virus-infected cells that are the targets of immune killer cells, which can eliminate the virus-infected cells. Doherty and Zinkernagel based their "altered self" or "dual recognition" theory on the observation that killer cells from virus-infected animals could only kill virus-infected cells in vitro if these cells carried the same H-2D or H-2K antigens as the infected animal in which the killer cells had been educated. This theory has now received substantial support from many other experiments and the same mechanism seems to work not only for virus antigens but also for many other antigens [20]. Although the details of the mechanism are still unknown, the scheme illustrated in Figure 2 seems to be compatible with most observations. The ABC antigens play a role by combining with foreign antigens and then presenting these in an "appetizing" form to immunocompetent lymphocytes. These lymphocytes are then triggered by the "altered" ABC antigens to develop into effector cells which can kill cells carrying the same foreign antigen complexed with the same ABC antigens. In other words the ABC antigens present foreign antigens to immunocompetent cells, which see the foreign antigen in combination with the ABC specificities.

The Ia antigens seemed not to play a similar role in Doherty and Zinkernagel's experiments with virus-infected cells. There is increasing evidence, however, that the Ia antigens also can present foreign antigens to immunocompetent cells [21–23]. In contrast to the relationship between ABC antigens and precursor T killer lymphocytes, Ia antigens present foreign antigens to other T cells, eg T helper lymphocytes which are generally necessary for B lymphocytes to transform into antibody-secreting cells. According to this model, the Ir genes may be identical to Ia genes, and there is no need to consider Ir determinants as immunoglobulin-like structures. Nevertheless, the Ir determinants must show some specificity, but even if, as we would like to think, Ia and Ir determinants are indeed present on the same molecule, it is completely unknown whether the Ia alloantigenic determinants are also responsible for the Ir function.

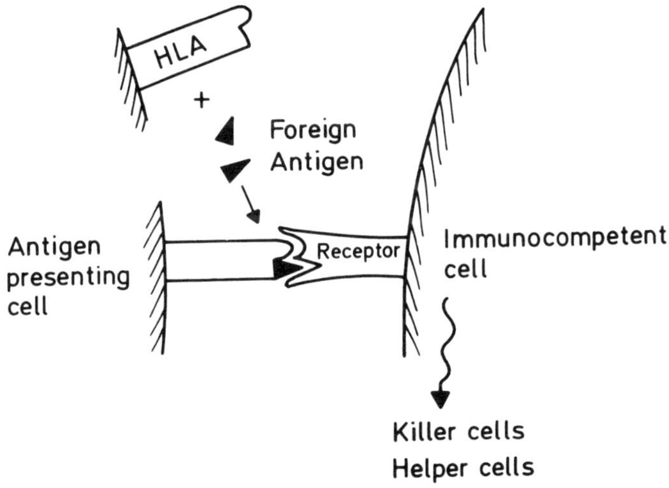

Fig. 2. Simplified model of "altered self." HLA antigen combines with foreign antigen and presents to immunocompetent lymphocytes, which transform into killer, helper or suppressor cells reactive with the foreign antigen only when it is presented by the same HLA antigen. Conceivably, some HLA antigens may be better suited than others in the presentation of a given foreign antigen.

HLA AND DISEASE

The strong interest evoked by the discovery of the HLA system was based on the assumption that this was the major histocompatibility system in man, and this assumption has now become an established fact: Kidneys transplanted from an HLA-identical (and ABO blood-group compatible) sib have a one-year survival rate of about 90%, and successful bone marrow transplantation has not been achieved across the HLA (more specifically the HLA-D) barrier.

The HLA system also plays a significant role in blood transfusion therapy. For example, febrile transfusion reactions, the most common untoward transfusion reactions, are mostly due to the destruction of donor granulocytes by preformed HLA alloantibodies in the recipient. Although unpleasant, these reactions are rarely dangerous and can be avoided by the use of leukocyte-poor blood. In thrombocytopenic patients who have developed HLA antibodies as the result of previous transfusions and/or pregnancies, successful platelet substitution can only be achieved with platelets from HLA-compatible donors.

At the time of writing, however, the most fascinating medical aspect of the HLA system seems to be its importance in relation to the susceptibility to a variety of diseases. The rest of this section will be devoted to these phenomena.

HLA and Disease Susceptibility

HLA had barely been recognized as a genetic system when Amiel postulated an association between a certain HLA antigen and Hodgkin disease [24]. It took many studies and many years before this association was confirmed. The first convincing associations of HLA and disease were reported in 1972, when psoriasis [25] and celiac disease [26] were found to be strongly associated with HLA-B13 and Bw17, and HLA-B8, respectively. The following year, the strongest association yet observed concerned the association between B27 and ankylosing spondylitis [27, 28]. The relationship between HLA and disease susceptibility has been the subject of several recent surveys [29–31] that discuss each disease in great detail with complete references. Here we will list the results of these numerous studies, and discuss their implications in diagnosis, nosology, and pathogenesis. Then we will present our understanding of the inheritance of disease susceptibility and mention some of the mechanisms which might explain these associations.

First, however, a few remarks are in order about how the studies are done and about some statistical problems. The easiest and most common approach is to study the frequencies of HLA antigens in a group of unrelated patients with the disease in question and compare them with the corresponding frequencies in a matched control group. One of the main difficulties of such population studies derives from the fact that about 20–25 different HLA antigens are usually determined and on a statistical basis there is a considerable probability that one or more of these will differ significantly between patients and controls by chance alone. This difficulty can be overcome by using more conservative probability levels before accepting an association as being biologically meaningful. A second problem is that even if a disease is related to HLA, this relationship may go undetected if typing for the HLA factor involved is not included in the study. Family studies can overcome this difficulty because the disease will then segregate with certain haplotypes within families. The drawback here is that in general only families with at least two affected relatives are informative.

The vast majority of the results collected so far derive from population studies. Table 2 summarizes our present knowledge in this regard [32]. For each disease, we have given the antigen(s) deviating from normal, the so-called "relative risk(s)," and the frequencies of the antigen(s) in patients and controls. The relative risk is a measure of the strength of the association and indicates how many times more frequently the disease occurs in individuals carrying the antigen than in individuals lacking the antigen. For example, ankylosing spondylitis is about 90 times more frequent in HLA-B27-positive than in B27-negative whites.

In many cases more than one antigen (often from different series) show association. In general, however, we have given in Table 2 only the results for the antigens showing the strongest association, since most of the other associations are probably due to linkage disequilibrium or allelic relationship between the corresponding HLA genes. It should be kept in mind, however, that HLA-D (and C) antigens have been studied much less often than A and B antigens. Accordingly, it is possible that some of the diseases listed in Table 2 as HLA-B-associated may be more strongly associated with HLA-D than with the antigens shown.

Diagnostic value. The high frequency (90%) of HLA-B27 in patients with ankylosing spondylitis compared to controls (9%) is already gaining increasing use in the diagnosis of this disorder, and it may be considered similar in value to the Waaler-Rose test in rheumatoid arthritis. Nevertheless, it should be kept in mind that HLA typing is rather expensive and that B27 cannot distinguish between ankylosing spondylitis, Reiter disease, or other reactive arthropathies. For most other conditions associated with HLA, diagnostic value of HLA typing seems small at the present time, but this situation could change when Ia-typing becomes better established.

Nosology. One important implication of the associations between HLA and disease is the opportunity now to reevaluate previous subdivisions of diseases and perhaps to establish new subdivisions. For example, the previously much debated distinction between juvenile and maturity-onset diabetes mellitus has been confirmed by the observation that only the juvenile (or rather the insulin-"dependent") form is associated with HLA, while the maturity-onset form is not. Another

TABLE 2. Associations Between HLA and Disease

Disease	HLA antigen	No. of studies	Frequency (%) Patients[a]	Frequency (%) Controls[b]	Relative risk	P-value[c]
RHEUMATOLOGY						
Ankylosing spondylitis						
Whites	B27	21	89	8.6	90.1	< 1E-10
Japanese	B27	2	77	1	324.5	< 1E-10
American blacks	B27	1	48	2	36.5	8.5E-07
American Indians	B27	1	100	51	34.4	1.7E-05
Reiter disease						
B27		8	77	8.6	35.9	< 1E-10
Yersinia arthritis						
B27		2	62	8.6	17.6	< 1E-10
Salmonella arthritis						
B27		2	62	8.6	17.6	3.6E-10
Psoriatic arthritis						
B27		5	45	8.6	8.6	< 1E-10
Juvenile rheumatoid arthritis						
B27		8	30	8.6	4.5	< 1E-10
Acute anterior uveitis						
B27		3	47	8.6	9.4	< 1E-10
Rheumatoid arthritis						
White	Dw4	1	45	17	3.9	5.5E-04
Mixed	Dw4	1	72	13	16.8	1.5E-08
NEUROLOGY						
Multiple sclerosis						
Dw2		7	57	23.6	4.3	< 1E-10
Optic neuritis						
Dw2		2	47	23.6	2.9	6.9E-05

Myasthenia gravis					
B8	5	58	23.7	4.4	< 1E-10
Dw3	2	38	21.0	2.3	5.6E-03
Paralytic poliomyelitis					
Bw16	2	20	5.4	4.3	2.9E-06
PSYCHIATRY					
Schizophrenia					
A28	5	20	10.0	2.3	3.9E-05
Manic depressive disorder					
Bw16	5	12	5.4	2.3	6.0E-05
DERMATOLOGY					
Psoriasis vulgaris					
B13	8	17	4.3	4.7	< 1E-10
Bw17	8	28	7.7	4.7	< 1E-10
Bw37	3	12	2.1	6.4	7.3E-08
Pustular psoriasis					
B27	2	26	8.6	3.7	1.8E-04
Dermatitis herpetiformis					
B8	7	73	23.7	8.7	< 1E-10
Dw3	2	78	21.0	13.5	< 1E-10
Pemphigus					
A10	4	23	9.6	2.8	1.5E-04
Behcet disease					
B5	5	47	10.6	7.4	< 1E-10
Recurrent herpes labialis					
A1	1	63	31.1	3.7	1.3E-08
B8	1	44	23.7	2.5	3.5E-04
Alopecia areata					
B12	1	55	25.2	3.6	2.6E-04

TABLE 2. Associations Between HLA and Disease (Continued)

Disease HLA antigen	No. of studies	Frequency (%) Patients[a]	Frequency (%) Controls[b]	Relative risk	P-value[c]
ENDOCRINOLOGY					
Juvenile diabetes					
B8	13	43	23.7	2.4	< 1E-10
B18	12	11	7.1	1.7	1.3E-06
Bw15	13	29	17.9	1.9	< 1E-10
Dw3	1	50	21.0	3.8	3.0E-04
Dw4	1	42	17.2	3.5	5.6E-05
Graves disease					
B8	7	42	23.7	2.3	< 1E-10
Dw3	2	54	21.0	4.4	4.9E-09
Idiopathic Addison disease					
B8	2	55	23.7	3.9	7.3E-06
Dw3	1	70	21.0	8.8	3.4E-07
Subacute thyroiditis					
Bw35	3	72	13.1	16.8	< 1E-10
Adrenocortical hyperfunction					
A1	1	53	31.1	2.5	9.4E-05
A3	1	10	26.9	0.29	9.5E-05

GASTROENTEROLOGY					
Celiac disease					
B8	11	73	23.7	8.6	< 1E-10
Dw3	1	95	21.0	73.0	< 1E-10
Pernicious anemia					
B7	6	38	26.8	1.7	4.5E-04
Autoimmune chronic hepatitis					
B8	8	47	23.7	2.9	< 1E-10
Dw3	1	64	21.0	6.8	3.2E-06
Idiopathic hemochromatosis					
A3	2	75	26.9	8.3	< 1E-10
B14	1	30	4.5	9.2	3.1E-06
IMMUNOPATHOLOGY					
Systemic lupus erythematosus					
B5	6	18	10.6	1.8	5.8E-05
B8	8	40	23.7	2.1	< 1E-10
Sicca syndrome					
B8	4	49	23.7	3.1	2.5E-10
Dw3	1	83	21.0	19.0	4.1E-08
MALIGNANT DISEASE					
Hodgkin disease					
A1	17	39	31.1	1.4	5.1E-08
B5	17	16	10.6	1.6	3.7E-07
B8	17	29	23.7	1.3	5.3E-05
B18	12	12	7.1	1.9	7.0E-08

TABLE 2. Associations Between HLA and Disease (Continued)

Disease HLA antigen	No. of studies	Frequency (%) Patients[a]	Controls[b]	Relative risk	P-value[c]
OTHER DISEASES					
Congenital heart malformation					
A2	1	85	53.6	4.9	1.3E-06
Polycystic kidney disease					
B5	2	24	10.6	2.6	2.5E-04
Appendicitis acuta					
B5	1	7	10.6	0.68	1.7E-04
B12	1	40	25.2	2.0	6.2E-10
B27	1	4	8.6	0.47	2.8E-05
Asbetosis					
B27	2	26	8.6	3.7	2.8E-04
Cryptogenic fibrosing alveolitis					
B12	1	76	25.2	9.4	1.1E-04

[a]The frequencies in patients have been calculated from the control frequencies and the combined estimates of relative risk. Data from Svejgaard and Ryder (1977) [32].

[b]The HLA frequencies in controls refer to a Danish population [31].

[c]P-values indicate the statistical significance of the deviations of the relative risks from unity and are given in floating-point notation, eg 6.9E-05 means 6.9×10^{-5}. The P-values have not been multiplied by the number of antigens studied.

example is psoriasis vulgaris, which can be separated from pustular psoriasis because the former is associated with HLA-B13, Bw17, and Bw37, whereas pustular psoriasis is not. Moreover, the HLA association with psoriasis vulgaris seems mainly, if not exclusively, to exist when the disease is diagnosed before the middle of the third decade. An analogous situation is that HLA-B8 associated with myasthenia gravis is mainly confined to women with early age at onset, without a thymoma, and without autoantibodies.

On the other hand, these associations can also be useful in grouping certain diseases. For example, the increase of HLA-B27 in ankylosing spondylitis, Reiter disease, and other reactive arthropathies, as well as in acute anterior uveitis and balanitis, confirms the relationship previously found between these conditions in clinical studies. The same is true for optic neuritis and multiple sclerosis, which are both associated with HLA-Dw2. Some organ-specific autoimmune diseases [33] can be grouped due to the association with Dw3 (eg insulin-dependent diabetes, Graves disease, and idiopathic Addison disease). In contrast, although they have been considered to belong to the organ-specific autoimmune group, Hashimoto thyroiditis and pernicious anemia are apparently not associated with the Dw3 antigen.

Inheritance of disease susceptibility. For most, but not all, of the diseases listed in Table 2, it has long been known that there is a tendency for a given disorder to occur with increased frequency in first-degree relatives (ie parents, sibs, and children) of affected individuals compared to the frequency of the disorder in the general population. This has been taken as evidence that genetic factors play a role in disease susceptibility, and additional support for this assumption has usually been obtained when twin studies have been carried out and revealed that there is a higher concordance rate in monozygotic than in dizygotic twins. The latter evidence weighs more strongly in terms of heredity than the former because relatives usually share, in addition to genetic factors, more environmental circumstances than unrelated individuals. The associations observed between these diseases and HLA finally proved that genetic factors are involved, and in addition they provide a tool to investigate the mode of inheritance of disease susceptibility which has previously remained very much in the dark: It was clearly neither simple dominant nor recessive. The diseases have often been said to be multifactorial, ie due to both genetic and environmental factors. The genetic part has usually been called polygenic [34, 35], ie due to many different genes at many loci. Each of these genes is believed to bring the individual closer to the threshold beyond which the disease develops under appropriate environmental conditions. Polygenic inheritance has often been considered as opposed to the results of a single gene with major effect, but as pointed out by Edwards [36], lack of penetrance and varying age at onset makes it extremely difficult to distinguish between these two models. Below we shall illustrate with some examples how the HLA and disease associations may help us to explore the heredity in more detail.

The HLA antigens are inherited characters associated with the diseases, but it is important to stress that the antigens indicated for the various diseases listed in Table 2 may not be the HLA factors truly responsible for disease susceptibility. The HLA system probably contains many more genes than those known today; it is possible that one or more of these as yet unknown HLA genes are involved, but if so they must be in linkage disequilibrium with those coding for the antigens now known to be associated. However, even with this reservation in mind, it is still possible to gain important insight into the mode of inheritance of the associated diseases.

Previous family studies of ankylosing spondylitis [34] have given results compatible with a polygenic inheritance for this disorder. However, the fact that about 90% of the patients are B27-positive as compared to about 9% of controls shows clearly that B27 (or another HLA gene closely associated with B27) is a gene of major effect as regards ankylosing spondylitis. Moreover, the mere observation that HLA-B27 heterozygous individuals have about the same risk of developing the disorder as B27 homozygotes indicates that the disease susceptibility is dominant even if it is not caused by the B27 antigen itself. In fact, mathematical analysis of the association strongly supports this assumption [37, 38]. The fact that the association with B27 holds for all races investigated (whites, American Indians, American blacks, and Japanese) provides evidence, but not proof, that it is B27 itself that confers the susceptibility to ankylosing spondylitis. If this is true, the observation that about 10% of ankylosing spondylitis patients are B27-negative indicates that the disease can develop without HLA involvement. It is worth noting that the frequency of B27 is approximately the same in female and in male patients, although the disease is quite strongly influenced by sex, being about five times more frequent in males than in females. It is of interest to note that investigations of "healthy" B27-positive individuals have revealed that about 25% of them show evidence of ankylosing spondylitis [37] indicating that this disorder is more frequent than has previously been suggested (this is particularly true for females).

The inheritance of diabetes mellitus has been the subject of many studies in the past, all of them inconclusive. The association between HLA and insulin-dependent diabetes has now thrown some light on the situation for this subgroup of the disease. At least five different antigens are increased in insulin-dependent diabetes: HLA-B8, B18, and Bw15 from the B series, and HLA-Dw3 and Dw4 from the D series. The increases of B8 and Bw15 are most probably secondary to the increases of Dw3 and Dw4, respectively [39], but many fewer patients have been studied for HLA-D than for HLA-A and B. As reported elsewhere [32, 39], the risk of diabetes is about twice as high for HLA-B8/w15 heterozygous than for individuals carrying only one of these antigens whether they are homozygous or not. We have taken this as evidence that there are two different HLA genes (in linkage disequilibrium with B8 and Bw15 respectively), which confer an increased risk of diabetes each by its own mechanism. When the two genes come together in the same individual they interact to further increase the disease susceptibility. Studies of families with two affected sibs have shown that there is an excess of HLA identity among these pairs [39], and this has been taken as evidence that the HLA-associated disease susceptibility is recessive [38]; however, this observation may equally well be explained by an over dominant action of two different HLA genes.

In psoriasis vulgaris, the situation is quite different: Here the risk of the disease is not influenced by the simultaneous occurrence of any of the three HLA-B antigens associated with this disease [31]. Accordingly, it is possible that there is only one HLA-linked gene conferring susceptibility to psoriasis, and as reported elsewhere [30], it is possible that this gene belongs to the C locus. The disease susceptibility is probably dominant as there is no increased risk for homozygotes.

Mechanisms explaining the associations. There are quite a number of different models that can explain why certain HLA factors confer susceptibility to disease [20, 31, 40–43].

For most of the diseases in Table 2, it seems most likely that the associations are due to the action of immune response determinants. Naturally, this is particularly true when the HLA-D or Ia antigens show the strongest associations. As discussed elsewhere [42], immune response determinants may influence disease susceptibility in various ways, eg via the generation of helper cells – or suppressor cells – directed against a specific antigen or group of antigens. These may be foreign antigens or self-antigens, and the disease process may involve decreased or excessive immunity to a foreign pathogen and/or autoimmunity.

With the discovery that HLA-ABC (and perhaps the Ia) antigens are involved in the "altered self" mechanism, it is also easy to envisage how these antigens could confer disease susceptibility. For example, a certain HLA antigen may have a particular affinity for, and be especially fit to present a viral antigen to, immunocompetent lymphocytes. This could lead to an overproduction of killer cells, which would kill not only virus-infected but perhaps also uninfected cells that have absorbed viral antigens to their HLA antigens.

Molecular mimicry is another theory according to which a microorganism possessing antigens resembling some HLA antigens may escape recognition by the immune system in individuals carrying these HLA antigens. However, it is perhaps more plausible that such molecular mimicry may result in breakdown of self-tolerance and consequent autoimmunity in such individuals. In any case, there is as yet little evidence of immunologic cross-reactivity between microbial and HLA antigens, but this possibility is far from having been exhaustively studied.

It is generally accepted that a virus must react with a receptor on the cell surface before it can infect the cell; it has also been suggested that HLA antigens may act as receptors for virus, but there is no evidence supporting this assumption at the present time.

Deficiency of the second component of complement (C2) is strongly associated with HLA-Dw2 and B18 and seems to be accompanied by an increased susceptibility to lupoid-like syndrome, but this condition apparently comprises so small a part of the lupoid spectrum that no association seems to exist between B18 and lupus erythematosus (Dw2 has not been studied).

The Ia antigens are so-called differentiation antigens both in the sense that they are primarily present on some cell types in the body and in the more extended meaning of this term, as they are involved in the cooperation between monocytes and T lymphocytes. The possibility that HLA may be involved in cellular differentiation at an earlier level has recently received some support by the observation that the Kostmann syndrome, a developmental defect of neutropoiesis, seems to be strongly associated with HLA-B12 [44].

Finally, in order to explain the associations between HLA and schizophrenia, manic depressive disease, and hemochromatosis, which do not seem to be due to "aberrant" immunity, the present authors have advanced the hypothesis [43] that HLA antigens may interfere with the reaction between hormones (or other ligands, eg neurotransmitters) and their receptors on the cell surface. The H-2 system of mice influences the concentration of testosterone in the blood [45] and of cyclic AMP in liver cells [46], and the recent observation of Yamazaki and co-workers [47] that mice show preferential mating according to their H-2 types further illustrates that these genetic systems also play a role outside the field of immunology.

What Is the Reason for the Diversity of the HLA System?

It is easy to understand that the immunoglobulins must show an enormous diversity in order to deal with the multitude of foreign antigens. How the diversity arises is still a matter of debate [48, 49]. In contrast, the origin of the diversity of the HLA system is easier to understand, since there have been mutations and gene duplications through many generations. The question is: Why is HLA so polymorphic? Indeed, the parallel between immunoglobulins and HLA is only superficial: The diversity of immunoglobulins is mainly intraindividual, while that of HLA is to a large extent interindividual.

Genetic polymorphism as defined by Ford [50] is the existence in a population of at least two alleles at a locus, each with a frequency higher than can be accounted for by the occurrence of new mutations. Ford estimated the lowest allele frequency of a polymorphic trait to be about 1% and suggested that special mechanisms would have to operate for traits exceeding this frequency. Some of the mechanisms maintaining polymorphism, among others, could be natural selection, genetic drift, or population stratification.

There must have been (and probably still is) a considerable freedom of mutations within the HLA system, since there are so many different alleles at each locus, and since none of these are incompatible with life. Then why have most of these alleles reached frequencies well above 1%? It seems unlikely to us that this pronounced polymorphism could be due solely to neutral mechanisms. Natural selection must have played a role.

Assuming that the biologic function of the HLA system is to act as the first frontier in the immune response against foreign organisms, it would seem advantageous for each individual to possess all the HLA factors necessary to combat all the dangerous microorganisms of the environment. Allowing for the possibility that there are probably several HLA isotypes shared by most human beings, it would appear that the advantages provided by the HLA polymorphism should probably be viewed in relation to the entire population rather than to the single individual. With many HLA alleles segregating in the population, there is a good possibility that at least some individuals of the group can effectively combat microorganism A and others microorganism B, etc. This is a so-called frequency-dependent selection. Naturally, this is not as effective a mechanism as if all individuals had all of the antigens. In that case, each subject would be resistant to all microorganisms; as it is now, several different microorganisms could eradicate the entire population by infecting it simultaneously or one after the other. Why then, do we not carry all the HLA antigens? One answer would be that there has not yet been time enough for sufficient gene duplications to occur. This is rather unlikely, considering the fact that these genetic systems show pronounced polymorphism in all vertebrates so far investigated. If it had been advantageous for each individual to carry many of these histocompatibility antigens, sufficient gene duplications should have taken place and become fixed in at least one of these species. Accordingly, in a teleogic sense, one is led to assume that it would be a disadvantage for the individual to carry more HLA antigens than he/she does. Conceivably, the presence of more HLA antigens would shift the balance from protection against microorganisms to susceptibility to autoimmunity and other disorders. In fact, Ceppellini [51] reported a tetragametic human who carried a double set of HLA antigens and suffered from several endocrine disorders. It is perhaps in this relation we should see the associations between HLA and disease. Most of the relationships described so far seem to confer dominant susceptibility to disease mostly of autoimmune nature. It is possible that these susceptibility factors (HLA-Dw3 in particular?) have been particularly effective against a range of microorganisms in the past, but that with changed environment, effective chemotherapy, and increasing life span of susceptible individuals, these genes display an adverse effect resulting in autoimmune-like phenomena rather than the protection against infection.

ACKNOWLEDGMENTS

We are grateful to Dr. Gary Troup and our colleagues at the laboratory for critical discussions, and to Ms. Elly Andersen and Ms. Elisabeth Schacht for expert secretarial assistance.

REFERENCES

1. Landsteiner K: Uber Agglutinationsercheinungen normalden menschlichen Blutes. Wien Klin Wochenschr 14:1132–1134, 1901.
2. Levine P, Stetson RE: An unusual case of intragroup agglutination. JAMA 113:126–127, 1939.
3. Marsh WL: Chronic granulomatous disease, the McLeod syndrome, and the Kell blood groups. This volume.
4. Dausset J: Isoleuco-anticorps. Acta Haematol 20:156–166, 1958.
5. Doherty PC, Zinkernagel RM: A biological role for the major histocompatibility antigens. Lancet 1:1406–1409, 1975.
6. McDevitt HO, Benacerraf B: Genetic control of specific immune response. Adv Immunol 11:31–74, 1969.
7. Ceppellini R, Curtoni ES, Mattiuz PL, Miggiano V, Scudeller G, Serra A: Genetics of leukocyte antigens: A family study of segregation and linkage. In "Histocompatibility Testing, 1967." Copenhagen: Munksgaard, 1967, pp 149–185.
8. Transplantation proceedings. Proc 6th Int Congr Transplant Soc 9, 1977.
9. Bodmer WF: HLA: A super supergene. Harvey Lect 1976/77 (In press).
10. Kissmeyer-Nielsen F (ed): "Histocompatibility Testing 1975." Copenhagen: Munksgaard, 1975.
11. Snell GD, Dausett J, Nathenson S: "Histocompatiblity." New York: Academic Press, 1976.
12. Svejgaard A, Hauge M, Jersild C, Platz P, Ryder LP, Nielsen LS, Thomsen M: "The HLA System. An Introductory Survey." In Beckman L, Hauge M (eds): Monographs in Human Genetics. Basel: S Karger, vol 7, 1975.
13. Terasaki PI, McClelland JD: Microdroplet assay of human serum cytotoxins. Nature 204:998–1000, 1964.
14. Francke U, Pellegrino MA: Assignment of the major histocompatibility complex to a region of the short arm of human chromosome 6. Proc Natl Acad Sci USA 74:1147–1151, 1977.
15. Lamm LU, Friedrich U, Petersen GB, Jørgensen J, Nielsen J, Therkelsen AJ, Kissmeyer-Nielsen F: Assignment of the major histocompatibility complex to chromosome No. 6 in a family with a pericentric inversion. Hum Hered 24:273–284, 1974.
16. Albrechtsen D, Solheim BG, Thorsby E: Serologic recognition of HLA-D-associated determinants. Transplant Proc 9:435–437, 1977.

17. van Rood JJ, van Leeuwen A, Keuning JJ, Blussé van Oud Alblas A: The serological recognition of the human MLC determinants using a modified cytotoxicity technique. Tissue Antigens 5:73–79, 1975.
18. Jersild C, Rubinstein P, Good RA, Day NK: The HLA system and inherited deficiencies of the complement system. Transplant Rev 32:43–71, 1976.
19. Bodmer WF, Thomson T: Population genetics and evolution of the HLA system. In Dausset J, Svejgaard A (eds): "HLA and Disease." Copenhagen: Munksgaard, 1977.
20. Zinkernagel RM, Doherty PC: Possible mechanisms of disease susceptibility association with major transplantation antigens. Ibid.
21. Cunningham AJ, Lafferty KJ: A simple conservative explanation of the H-2 restriction of interactions between lymphocytes. Scand J Immunol 6:1–6, 1977.
22. Rosenthal AS, Barcinski MA, Blake JT: Determinant selection is a macrophage-dependent immune response gene function. Nature 267:156–158, 1977.
23. Zinkernagel RM, Althage A, Adler B, Blanden RV, Davidson WF, Kees U, Dunlop MBC, Shreffler DC: H-2 restriction of cell-mediated immunity to an intracellular bacterium: Effector T cells are specific for Listeria antigen in association with H-21 region-coded self-markers. J Exp Med 145:1353–1367, 1977.
24. Amiel JF: Study of the leucocyte phenotypes in Hodgkin's disease. In "Histocompatibility Testing." Copenhagen: Munksgaard, 1967, pp 79–81.
25. Russell TJ, Schultes LM, Kuban DJ: Histocompatibility (HL-A) antigens associated with psoriasis. N Engl J Med 287:738–739, 1972.
26. Falchuk ZM, Rogentine GN, Strober W: Predominance of histocompatibility antigen HL-A8 in patients with gluten-sensitive enteropathy. J Clin Invest 51:1602–1605, 1972.
27. Brewerton DA, Caffrey M, Hart FD, James DCO, Nicholls A, Sturrock RD: Ankylosing spondylitis and HL-A27. Lancet 1:904–907, 1973.
28. Schlosstein L, Terasaki PI, Bluestone R, Pearson CM: High association of an HL-A antigen, W27, with ankylosing spondylitis. N Engl J Med 288:704–706, 1973.
29. Dausset J, Svejgaard A (eds): "HLA and Disease." Copenhagen: Munksgaard, 1977.
30. Ryder LP, Svejgaard A: Histocompatibility associated disease. In Loor F, Roelants GE (eds): "T and B Lymphocytes in Immune Responses." New York: Wiley, 1977, pp 437–456.
31. Svejgaard A, Platz P, Ryder LP, Nielsen LS, Thomsen M: HL-A and disease associations – A survey. Transplant Rev 22:3–43, 1975.
32. Svejgaard A, Ryder LP: Associations between HLA and disease. Notes on methodology and a report from the HLA and disease registry. In Dausset J, Svejgaard A (eds): "HLA and Disease." Copenhagen: Munksgaard, 1977.
33. Nerup J: Addison's disease. A review of some clinical, pathological and immunological features. Dan Med Bull 21:201, 1974.
34. Carter CO: Genetics of common disorders. Br Med Bull 25:52–57, 1969.
35. Cavalli-Sforza LL, Bodmer WF: "The Genetics of Human Populations." San Francisco: WH Freeman, 1971.
36. Edwards JH: Familial predisposition in man. Br Med Bull 25:58–64, 1969.
37. Kidd KK, Bernoco D, Carbonara AO, Daneo V, Steiger U, Ceppellini R: Genetic analysis of HLA associated diseases: The 'illness susceptible' gene frequency and sex ratio in ankylosing spondylitis. In Dausset J, Svejgaard A (eds): "HLA and Disease." Copenhagen: Munksgaard, 1977.
38. Thomson G, Bodmer W: The genetic analysis of HLA and disease associations. Ibid.

39. Nerup J, Cathelineau C, Seignalet J, Thomsen M: HLA and endocrine diseases. Ibid.
40. McDevitt HO, Bodmer WF: HL-A, immune response genes and disease. Lancet 1:1269–1275, 1974.
41. Snell GD: The H-2 locus of the mouse. Observation and speculations concerning its comparative genetics and its polymorphism. Folia Biol (Praha) 14:335–358, 1968.
42. Svejgaard A, Platz P, Ryder LP: Associations between HLA and some non-rheumatic diseases and possible explanations. In Brewerton DA (ed): "Immunogenetics and Rheumatic Disease." Clinics in Rheumatic Disease, 1977. Vol 13, pp 239–253.
43. Svejgaard A, Ryder LP: Interaction of HLA molecules with non-immunological ligands as an explanation of HLA and disease associations. Lancet 2:547–549, 1976.
44. Hansen JA, Dupont B, L'Esperance P, Good RA: Congenital neutropenia: Abnormal neutrophil differentiation associated with HLA. Immunogenetics 4:327–332, 1977.
45. Iványi P, Forejt J: Genetic factors closely associated with the major histocompatibility system: Structural and/or regulatory genes. In Libansky J, Donner L (eds): "Present Problems in Haematology." Amsterdam–Prague: Excerpta Medica and Avicenum, 1974, p 143.
46. Meruelo D, Edidin M: Association of mouse liver adenosine 3′,5′-cyclic monophosphate (cyclic AMP) levels with histocompatibility-2 genotype (cell-surface/polypeptide hormones/h-2 antigens). Proc Natl Acad Sci USA 72:2644–2648, 1975.
47. Yamazaki K, Boyse EA, Miké V, Thaler HT, Mathieson BJ, Abbott J, Boyse J, Zayas ZA, Thomas L: Control of mating preference in mice by genes in the major histocompatibility complex. J Exp Med 144:1324, 1976.
48. Jerne NK: The somatic generation of immune recognition. Eur J Immunol 1:1–9, 1971.
49. Wigzell H: Antibody diversity: Is it all coded for by the germ line genes? Scand J Immunol 2:199–206, 1973.
50. Ford EB: Polymorphism. Biol Rev 20:73–88, 1945.
51. Ceppellini R: Old and new facts and speculations about transplantation antigens of man. In Amos B (ed): "Progress in Immunology. First International Congress of Immunology." New York: Academic Press, 1971, pp 952–1025.

SECTION II:
THE IMMUNE DEFENSE SYSTEM

Normal T- and B-Cell Differentiation: Correlation With Defects Producing Immune Deficiency*

Alexander R. Lawton, MD, and Max D. Cooper, MD

INTRODUCTION

In using the term "experiments of nature" to characterize the congenital immune deficiencies, Dr. Robert Good has emphasized the immense potential of study of patients with these conditions for understanding the normal development of immunologic functions. The reverse is equally true: Knowledge of the cellular interactions which regulate development and function of the immune system, and of their controlling genetic mechanisms, will eventually provide the clues needed for understanding and treating these defects. Both sides of this coin are represented in the contents of this symposium. In this review we will describe briefly some recent observations on the morphologic and functional ontogeny of T and B lymphocytes, and attempt to illustrate relationships to some common forms of immunodeficiency.

DEVELOPMENT OF B CELLS

Genesis of B cells begins within the fetal liver by the 8th or 9th week of gestation, perhaps slightly earlier than T cells begin their development within the thymus. The immediate progenitor of both B and T cells is probably a lymphoid stem cell, which in turn is derived from a pluripotent hemopoietic stem cell. Convincing evidence for a separate lymphoid stem cell was recently provided by observations on women with polycythemia vera who were also

*Research from the authors' laboratories was supported by The National Foundation–March of Dimes grant 1–354, and by NIH grants AI 11502, CA 16673, CA 13148 and RR 32. Dr. Lawton is the recipient of NIH Research Career Development Award AI 70780.

Birth Defects: Original Article Series, Volume XIV, Number 6A, pages 49–57

heterozygous for X-linked isoenzymes of glucose-6-phosphate dehydrogenase. Cells of the myeloid, megakaryocytic, and erythroid lines expressed only one allele, while both were represented in lymphocytes [1].

The earliest B cell is a large, rapidly dividing lymphocyte which synthesizes IgM in small amounts. These cells, called pre-B, can be distinguished from conventional B lymphocytes by several criteria, the most important of which is the lack of expression of membrane-bound IgM (sIgM) in quantities sufficient to be detectable by immunofluorescence. Pre-B cells were first morphologically identified as cells containing small amounts of cytoplasmic IgM (cIgM) in liver of fetal mice, where they preceded development of sIgM+ B lymphocytes by several days [2]. During fetal life these cells can be found in various lymphoid tissues, but in adult mice, rabbits, and humans they persist only in the bone marrow. There is abundant evidence, both functional and morphologic, that the generative pool of pre-B cells gives rise to sIgM-positive B lymphocytes (reviewed in Lawton and Cooper [3]). As pre-B cells from rabbits heterozygous for co-dominant allelic forms of kappa light chains express one or the other alternative allotype [4], it is likely that the processes of gene selection involved in generation of diversity of antibody combining sites occur during this developmental stage. A by-product of the identification of pre-B cells, and of their restricted tissue distribution, is the very strong implication that fetal liver, and later adult bone marrow, serve as mammalian equivalents of the avian bursa.

Two additional characteristics are shared by immature B lymphocytes in fetal liver and adult bone marrow. As mentioned earlier, the earliest B lymphocytes which develop in human fetal liver at 9–10 weeks, or in the mouse at 16–17 days, bear only sIgM [2, 3]. These cells are functionally quite different from mature sIgM+ lymphocytes. Adult B lymphocytes, when treated in vitro with bivalent antibodies to IgM, for a period of time lose detectable sIgM. This phenomenon, called antigenic modulation, results from a series of energy-dependent events on the cell membrane through which complexes of receptor IgM and antibody form aggregates. These aggregates migrate to one pole of the cell (cap formation) and are then internalized by reverse pinocytosis [5]. Modulation of immature B lymphocytes differs in at least two important respects. First, it occurs at much lower concentrations of antibody than is needed to cause equivalent modulation of adult cells; second, subsequent to such treatment immature B lymphocytes fail to reexpress sIgM, while adult cells do so during 24 hours in culture [6, 7]. Similarly, development of B lymphocytes and plasma cells in vivo can be almost completely arrested by injections of anti-μ antibodies, but only if the treatment is begun very shortly after birth [8]. The biologic significance of these observations was brought into focus by Metcalf and

Klinman [9], who demonstrated that exposure of fetal or neonatal B lymphocytes to conventional multivalent antigens in the absence of appropriately primed T cells resulted in specific immunologic tolerance. The same populations stimulated with the same antigens, but in the presence of helper T cells, were entirely capable of generating an immune response. Finally, adult B cells were not affected at all in their response by prior exposure to antigens [9]. This unique susceptibility to tolerance wanes rapidly after birth, and is no longer demonstrable in spleen cells by the second week of life. The loss of tolerance susceptibility correlates closely with the rate of increase in resistance to supression of B-cell differentiation induced by lipopolysaccharide by anti-IgM antibodies [10]. The sensitivity of immature B lymphocytes to modulation, which is a property of human and chicken cells as well [11, 12], and to tolerance induction is shared by a portion of bone marrow B lymphocytes of adult mice [13], again suggesting that the marrow is a site of primary B-cell differentiation.

A third unique feature of fetal liver and adult marrow B lymphocytes relates to expression of the second major class of surface immunoglobulin, sIgD, on sIgM+ lymphocytes. In man, sIgD becomes detectable at about 12 weeks, or 3 weeks later than sIgM, and is expressed exclusively on sIgM+ cells. It is of interest that sIgG and sIgA appear either slightly earlier (IgG) or at about the same time, and these classes also are expressed only together with sIgM [3, 11]. Following its appearance sIgD rapidly becomes a major cell surface Ig, being present on 70–95% of sIgM+ cells in peripheral tissues. However, the proportion of sIgM+ cells which are also sIgD+ is characteristically low (< 50%) in fetal liver and adult bone marrow. It has been suggested that acquistion of sIgD may be the factor responsible for the loss of tolerance susceptibility of immature B cells [14]. Another important cell membrane component, Ia antigens encoded by genes in the immune response region of the major histocompatibility complex, might also be responsible for this change. The rate at which sIgM+ cells acquire Ia is more closely correlated with loss of tolerance susceptibility than is the rate of acquisition of sIgD [15].

The proportions of B lymphocytes in human lymphoid tissues increase rapidly, so that by 15 weeks gestation all classes are represented in adult proportions [16]. Recent studies indicate that the majority of B lymphocytes in one-week-old mice or neonatal humans [11] express multiple immunoglobulin classes. For example, the sequence of development of isotype expression on B cells becoming committed to IgA synthesis is likely: sIgM+ → sIgM+ · sIgA+ → sIgM+ · sIgA+ · sIgD+. These events occur independently of influences of antigen or of T cells, although it is clear that these factors may modify expression of class during subsequent differentiation. There is less secure evidence that multiple isotype expression is lost in reverse order during antigen-driven differentiation, with sIgD being lost first. In any case, the majority of circulating B lymphocytes in adult human blood which express sIgG or sIgA do not bear sIgM or sIgD. A more complete discussion of the development of B lymphocyte class diversity is presented elsewhere [17].

FUNCTIONAL ONTOGENY OF B-CELL RESPONSE IN MAN

Although the human fetus is capable of mounting an antibody response by about 20 weeks gestation [18], there are both quantitative and qualitative differences between fetal and adult antibody production. These differences may be seen in the development of serum immunoglobulins. IgM is normally present in neonatal blood at approximately 10% of the adult concentration, and reaches adult levels by 9–12 months. The capacity to synthesize IgG develops more slowly, and IgA lags even more; adult concentrations of the latter generally are acquired by the time of puberty. The delay in onset of production of IgG and IgA cannot be accounted for on the basis of late development of the relevant precursor B lymphocytes, since these are present by the end of the first trimester of fetal life.

The development of an in vitro technique for studying differentation of human B lymphocytes to plasma cells [19] allowed us to begin to study this problem. In our laboratory LYF Wu determined that the ontogeny of the capacity of lymphocytes from fetuses, infants, and young children to respond to pokeweed mitogen (PWM) with plasma cell differentiation closely mimicked the development of serum immunoglobulin concentrations. Fetal lymphocytes gave a meager response which was almost entirely restricted to the IgM class. Neonatal lymphocytes responded better, but rarely generated IgG or IgA plasma cells. The latter classes, and particularly IgA, were not regularly observed until after the first year [20].

The utility of the PWM assay for ontogenetic studies, and also for analysis of immune deficiences, was greatly enhanced with the discovery that T cells regulate this B-cell response. Waldman and co-workers showed that T cells from some hypogammaglobulinemic patients supressed the response of normal lymphocytes to PWM [21]. Janossy and Greaves [22] and Keightley et al [23] independently discovered that B lymphocytes deprived of T cells failed to proliferate or differentiate in response to PWM. Since allogeneic mixtures of normal T and B cells responded as well as unfractionate syngeneic lymphocytes to this mitogen, it became possible to independently assess T and B cell function [23].

Anthony Hayward has recently used these techniques in our laboratory to determine whether the defects observed earlier in the response of fetal or neonatal lymphocytes could be attributed to T cells or B cells or both [24]. Three sorts of experiments were done. First, fetal spleen cells were supplemented with adult T cells in order to determine whether their poor response was due to deficiencies in numbers or activity of T cells. Second, neonatal and adult peripheral lymphocytes were separated into T-and B-cell fractions and then cultured in all 4 possible combinations. Third, the possibility that neonatal T cells might suppress B cell differentiation was explored by adding various numbers of newborn or adult T cells to cultures containing a responding population of adult T and B cells.

The results of these experiments indicate involvement of at least 3 factors in the observed differences between fetal and adult response. As had been previously observed, fetal spleen cells responded poorly to PWM and produced a significant response only of the IgM class. Addition of adult "helper" T cells substantially increased the numbers of plasma cells formed, but failed to bring forth significant IgG or IgA responses. These results indicated that the poor response of fetal cells was partly due to deficiencies in number or activity of T cells, but also that the populations of sIgG+ and sIgA+ B lymphocytes present in fetal spleen were functionally immature. Somewhat different, but confirmatory, results were obtained with neonatal lymphocytes. Neonatal B cells cocultured with adult, as opposed to neonatal, T cells produced increased numbers of plasma cells of all 3 classes. In the reciprocal experiments, it was found that the substitution of neonatal for adult T cells substantially reduced the response of adult B cells. Moreover, while the IgM response dropped by an average of 50%, the IgG and IgA responses were diminished by 90%. Since adult T cells did not bring the responses of neonatal B cells to normal, it is again suggested that the latter are functionally immature. Also, however, neonatal T cells appear to be deficient with respect to their ability to support IgG and IgA responses by adult B cells.

Neonatal T cells were also found capable of suppressing the response of normal adult lymphocytes. This effect was highly variable in degree, but was found in 7 of 8 experiments, whereas addition of similar numbers of adult T cells to responding cultures never produced suppression. In only one instance did the magnitude of suppression approach that seen in some patients with hypogammaglobulinemia [21]. The finding of neonatal suppressor T-cell activity raised the question of whether the "decreased help" of neonatal T cells in the earlier experiments could be entirely due to "increased suppression." That this is probably not the case was suggested by the fact that neonatal suppressor cells diminished IgM, IgG, and IgA responses in parallel. On the other hand, in the assays for helper activity neonatal T cells were relatively effective in promoting IgM responses, but deficient in generating IgG or IgA plasma cells.

RELATIONSHIPS TO IMMUNODEFICIENCY

The preceding discussion of B-cell development has been written with the intent of illustrating some principles which may be applied to analyzing potential causes of some common immunodeficiencies. Primary B-cell differentiation is clearly a process which is genetically regulated; it begins in a specific anatomic site and at a specific time during embryogenesis; it proceeds through a series of distinct morphologic and functional stages leading from a few pluripotent stem cells to a vast number of competent lymphocytes, each committed to synthesize antibody molecules of a single specificity. A number of different factors are involved in regulation of B-cell differentiation. Primary differentiation of B cells occurs independent of the influence of antigen and of T cells, although each of these factors may modify the development of specific clones. For example, it is likely that clones of B lymphocytes recognizing "self" antigens are normally generated under influences of specific inductive microenvironments, and then may be eliminated by contact with those antigens during the stage when they are highly susceptible to being rendered tolerant.

The later stages of B-cell differentiation involve the conversion of small lymphocytes to antibody-secreting plasma cells. This process is dependent on contact with specific antigens and is regulated by interactions with macrophages and T lymphocytes. It is now clear that T cells are not a homogeneous population responsible for "cell-mediated immunity," but consist of several subsets of cells with distinct functional activities. Among these are "helper" T cells, which collaborate in the triggering of B-cell differentiation and "supressor" T cells which have precisely the opposite effect [25]. Studies in mice [26], as well as the experiments with neonatal cells described earlier, indicate that T cells carrying out these functions develop at different rates, so that suppressor activity dominates during fetal life. This activity may be critical to the maintenance of pregnancy. It has been shown that neonatal T cells can specifically inhibit proliferation of maternal lymphocytes, providing a mechanism by which the fetus could prevent an immunologic reaction of maternal cells against itself [27].

In 1971 it was demonstrated that patients with panhypogammaglobulinemia were heterogeneous with respect to the development of B lymphocytes [28]. It has since been determined that boys with congenital X-linked agammaglobulinemia have virtually no circulating B lymphocytes, while both male and female patients with equivalent deficiency of circulating immunoglobulins may have normal or only moderately decreased numbers of circulating B lymphocytes [29, 30].

These observations rather clearly demarcated two types of pathogenetic mechanisms in hypogammaglobulinemia. Deficiency of B lymphocytes must involve abnormalities of primary, antigen-independent, B-cell development. In contrast, the presence of normal numbers of B lymphocytes implies a lesion in the triggering mechanisms through which B lymphocytes, regulated by interactions with macrophages and T cells, are stimulated to plasma cell differentiation.

The definition of pre-B cells by ontogenetic studies provided a new means of dissecting primary B-cell deficiencies. In our laboratory Dr. Elliot Pearl has found that the frequency of pre-B cells in the marrow of boys with X-linked agammaglobulinemia (X-LA) is identical to that of normals. On the other hand, patients with acquired deficiency of B lymphocytes, included two individuals in which hypogammaglobulinemia is associated with thymoma, may have markedly reduced numbers of pre-B cells. It was mentioned earlier that patients with common variable hypogammaglobulinemia may have either normal or reduced numbers of B lymphocytes. In analyzing a group of such individuals, a highly significant correlation was found between the frequency of marrow pre-B cells and numbers of circulating B lymphocytes. This information permits further subdivision of patients with defects in primary B-cell development: boys with X-LA manifest a block in conversion of pre-B cells to mature B lymphocytes, while many patients with acquired deficiency of B lymphocytes apparently have an earlier lesion involving genesis of pre-B cells from their stem cell precursors [31].

Understanding the pathogenesis of B lymphocyte triggering defects requires functional assays capable of measuring the integrity of the cellular collaborations involved in terminal B-cell differentiation. One such technique, utilizing pokeweed mitogen as a T-dependent B-cell activator, was described above. By means of using this assay system a bewildering spectrum of abnormalities, ranging from excess suppressor T-cell activity [21] to intrinsic abnormalities of B lymphocytes [32] has been demonstated. It is particularly interesting that the types of abnormalities which have been found in patients are very similar to those described earlier as characteristic of normal ontogeny: B lymphocytes generated early in fetal life, particularly those destined to make IgG and IgA responses, are relatively incapable of being stimulated even in the presence of normal adult T cells; fetal and neonatal T cells apparently lack full competence as "helper" cells and have a relative excess of suppressor activity. These correlations carry the strong implication that more refined analysis of the molecular and genetic regulation of development of the immune system and of its subsequent function will provide the information necessary to understand, and to treat, an important group of birth defects.

REFERENCES

1. Adamson JW, Fialkow PJ, Murphy S, Prahl JF, Steinmann L: Polycythemia vera: Stem cell and probable clonal origin of the disease. N Engl J Med 295:913, 1976.
2. Raff MC, Megson M, Owen JJT, Cooper MD: Early production of intracellular IgM by B lymphocyte precursors in mouse. Nature 259:224, 1976.
3. Lawton AR, Cooper MD: Two new stages of antigen-independent B cell development in mice and humans. In Cooper MD, Dayton DH (eds): "Development of Host Defenses." Hewlett, NY: Raven Press (In press).
4. Hayward AR, Simon M, Lawton AR, Cooper MD, Mage RG: Pre-B cells and B cells in rabbits: Ontogeny and allelic exclusion. Fed Proc 36:1295, 1977.
5. Taylor RB, Duffus PH, Raff MC, dePetris S: Redistribution and pinocytosis of lymphocyte of surface immunoglobulin molecules induced by anti-immunoglobulin molecules. Nature (New Biol) 223:225, 1971.
6. Raff MC, Owen JJT, Cooper MD, Lawton AR, Megson M, Gathings WE: Differences in susceptibility of mature and immature mouse B lymphocytes to anti-immunoglobulin-induced immunoglobulin suppression in vitro: Possible implications for B cell tolerance to self. J Exp Med 142:1052, 1975.
7. Sidman CL, Unanue ER: Receptor-mediated inactivation of early B lymphocytes. Nature 257:149, 1975.
8. Lawton AR, Cooper MD: Modification of B lymphocyte differentiation by anti-immunoglobulins. In Cooper MD, Warner NL (eds): "Contemporary Topics in Immunobiology." vol 3. New York: Plenum, 1974, p 193.
9. Metcalf ES, Klinman NR: In vitro tolerance induction of neonatal murine B cells. J Exp Med 143:1327, 1976.
10. Kearney JF, Cooper MD, Lawton AR: Lymphocyte differentiation induced by lipopolysaccharide: III. Suppression of B cell maturation by anti-mouse immunoglobulin antibodies. J Immunol 116:1664, 1976.
11. Gathings WE, Lawton AR, Cooper MD: Lymphocyte studies of the development of pre-B cells, B lymphocytes and immunoglobulin isotype diversity in humans. Eur J Immunol (In press).
12. Grossi CE, Lydyard PM, Cooper MD: Ontogeny of B cells in the chicken. II. Changing patterns of cytoplasmic IgM expression and of modulation requirements for surface IgM by anti-μ antibodies. J Immunol (In press).
13. Metcalf ES, Klinman NR: In vitro tolerance induction of bone marrow cells: A marker for B cell maturation. J Immunol (In press).
14. Vitetta ES, Uhr J: Immunoglobulin receptors revisited. Science 189:964, 1975.
15. Kearney JF, Cooper MD, Klein J, Abney ER, Parkhouse RME, Lawton AR: Ontogeny of Ia and IgD on IgM-bearing B lymphocytes in mice. J Exp Med (In press).
16. Lawton AR, Self KS, Royal SA, Cooper MD: Ontogeny of B lymphocytes in the human fetus. Clin Immunol Immunopathol 1:104, 1972.
17. Cooper MD, Kearney JF, Lawton AR, Abney ER, Parkhouse RME, Preud'homme JL, Seligmann M: Generation of immunoglobulin class diversity in B cells: A discussion with emphasis on IgD development. Ann Immunol (Paris) 127:573, 1976.
18. Alford CA: Studies on antibody in congenital rubella infections. Am J Dis Child 110:455, 1965.
19. Wu LYF, Lawton AR, Cooper MD: Differentiation capacity of cultured B lymphocytes from immunodeficient patients. J Clin Invest 52:3180, 1973.
20. Wu LYF, Blanco A, Cooper MD, Lawton AR: Ontogeny of B lymphocyte differentiation induced by pokeweed mitogen. Clin Immunol Immunopathol 5:208, 1976.

21. Waldmann TA, Broder S, Blaese RM, Durm M, Blackman M, Strober W: Role of suppressor T cells in pathogenesis of common variable hypogammaglobulinemia. Lancet 2:609, 1974.
22. Janossy G, Greaves MF: Functional analysis of murine and human B lymphocyte subsets. Transplant Rev 24:177, 1975.
23. Keightley RK, Cooper MD, Lawton AR: The T cell dependence of B cell differentiation induced by pokeweed mitogen. J Immunol 117:1538, 1976.
24. Hayward AR, Lawton AR: Functional immaturity of human fetal lymphocytes. J Immunol (In press).
25. Katz DH: General resume of genetic requirements for cell-cell interactions. This volume pp 59–72.
26. Mosier DE, Johnson BM: Ontogeny of mouse lymphocyte function. II. Development of the ability to produce antibody is modulated by T lymphocytes. J Exp Med 141:216, 1975.
27. Olding LB, Benuschke K, Oldstone MBA: Inhibition of mitosis of lymphocytes from human adults by lymphocytes from human newborns. Clin Immunol Immunopathol 3:79, 1974.
28. Cooper MD, Lawton AR, Bockman DE: Agammaglobulinemia with B lymphocytes: Specific defect of plasma cell differentiation. Lancet 2:791, 1971.
29. Cooper MD, Keightley RG, Wu LYF, Lawton AR: Developmental defects of T and B cells in humans. Transplant Rev 16:51, 1973.
30. Preud'homme JL, Griscelli C, Seligmann M: Immunoglobulin on the surface of lymphocytes in fifty patients with primary immunodeficiency diseases. Clin Immunol Immunopathol 1:241, 1973.
31. Pearl ER, Vogler LB, Crist WM, Lawton AR, Cooper MD: Normal and aberrant B cell differentiation in bone marrow. Pediatr Res 11:491, 1977.
32. De La Coucha EG, Oldham G, Webster ADB, Asherson GL, Platts-Mills TAE: Quantitative measurements of T- and B-cell function in "variable" primary hypogammaglobulinemia: Evidence for a consistent B cell defect. Clin Exp Immunol 27:208, 1977.

Genetic Control of Cell-Cell Interactions in the Immune System*

David H. Katz, MD

The immune system is one of the most intricate of all body systems, paralleling in many respects the endocrine system in terms of the multiplicity of functions required of it for maintaining homeostasis and integrity of each individual's health. Both systems exert control over discreet functions at great distances within the body by virtue of circulating components capable of performing their role(s) at sites quite removed from their point(s) of origin, and in this sense they display a level of versatility not found in most other multicellular organ systems. They differ, however, in one important respect: The endocrine system encompasses several distinct endocrine organs each endowed with specific, and limited, functional capabilities; each organ is comprised of distinctive cell types in architecture, and the complexity of the system itself stems from the intricate communications network existing among these organs (and their respective target tissues) mediated in large part by their hormonal products generally unique to each of them. In contrast, the immune system consists of relatively few distinct organs – ie thymus, spleen, bone marrow, and lymph nodes – which are composed of relatively few distinct cell types. Although it is true that there are numerous lymph nodes throughout the body each one is generally structured in much the same manner as all the rest. In addition, lymph nodes appear to owe their multiplicity to the strategic nature of their different locations more so than any differences in general function.

Accordingly, the complexity of the immune system has evolved from an intriguing communications network established between the components of the system, designed in such a manner as to permit a multiplicity of effects to arise

*Studies performed in my laboratory have been supported by NIH grant AI-13874. This is publication number 38 from the Department of Cellular and Developmental Immunology and publication number 1346 from the Immunology Departments, Scripps Clinic and Research Foundation, La Jolla, California.

Birth Defects: Original Article Series, Volume XIV, Number 6A, pages 59–72

from relatively few distinct cell types. This has been accomplished by development of sophisticated regulatory mechanisms allowing either enormous amplification or contraction of a given response depending on the needs of the individual. Under normal circumstances, this system functions remarkably well to maintain effective defenses against foreign agents and against aberrant native cells which may have undergone neoplastic transformation either as a consequence of normal random mutational events or secondary to exogenous oncogenic influences. Many other circumstances exist, however, in which abnormalities in one or more components of the system result in some form of breakdown in the network manifested clinically in various ways and levels of severity.

In this presentation, I will emphasize essentially 2 major points: The first point is that the immune system is regulated by a series of complex cell-cell interactions which form the fundamental basis of an intricate communications network generally responsive to the needs of maintaining integrity of the individual. The second point is that such cell-cell interactions take place via a highly specific and sophisticated form of recognition events involving a large family of cell surface molecules encoded by genes located in a small chromosomal segment known as the major histocompatibility gene complex.

CELLS OF THE IMMUNE SYSTEM

As shown in Figure 1, the major cellular components of the immune system are the macrophages and lymphocytes. Macrophages are very versatile in the functions they perform in a variety of immune responses (see Ref. 1 for review). Although not themselves specific for any given antigen, they perform a crucial role in concentrating and presenting antigens to lymphocytes; in particular, they appear to determine, in some way, whether and which T lymphocytes will be stimulated by various antigens. Moreover, macrophages secrete several biologically active mediators capable of regulating the type and magnitude of lymphocyte responses by either enhancing or suppressing cell division and/or differentiation.

The lymphocytes represent the *specific* cellular component of the system, specificity being conferred upon such cells by virtue of the existence of antigen-specific receptors on the surface membrane of each immunocompetent cell. The nature of receptor specificity is highly specialized in that each different clone of lymphocytes expresses its own unique specificity. There are 2 major classes of lymphocytes; both classes ultimately derive from stem cells in the bone marrow. However, one class of lymphocytes is dependent upon hormonal influences of the thymus in order to undergo the very early stages of differentiation. These cells are therefore termed T lymphocytes. The other class of lymphocytes, known as B lymphocytes, undergo their major stages of differentiation in the absence

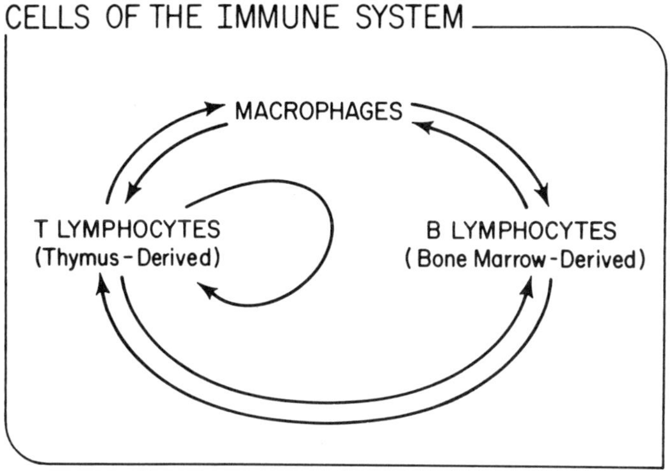

Fig. 1. From [22] reprinted with permission.

of any known influence of the thymus although, as will be discussed below, their final phases of differentiation in general are highly dependent upon the function of T lymphocytes.

In terms of surface antigen-specific receptors, it is well established that surface immunoglobulin (Ig) molecules serve as the antigen receptors for the B lymphocytes. The precise molecular nature of antigen receptors on T lymphocytes has not been definitively established, although recent data strongly indicate that at least one portion of the receptor molecule may be encoded by the very same genes encoding the combining site portion of conventional immunoglobulins [2, 3].

A major point to emphasize about the depiction of these cell types shown in Figure 1 is that the relationship between such cells, in the functional sense, is reciprocal and circumscribed. Thus, as indicated by the directional arrows, biologic activity of each respective cell type interplays in a complex fashion with each of the other cell types illustrated; this, indeed, forms the basis of the complex communication network that exists to regulate immunologic activity.

CELL-CELL INTERACTIONS IN THE IMMUNE SYSTEM

During the past decade, there have been several revolutionary conceptual developments in our understanding of cellular and molecular mechanisms involved in the functions of the immune system. This era was ushered in by the observations of Claman and his co-workers [4] which demonstrated that the development of antibody responses in certain instances required cooperative interactions between the 2 distinct classes of lymphocytes, namely T cells and B cells. These findings were subsequently confirmed and extended by others [5, 6] who furthermore documented that B cells were the actual precursors of antibody-forming cells while T cells provided an important, although undefined, auxiliary function necessary for B cell precursors to fully develop into mature antibody-secreting cells. Such observations therefore initiated the evolution of our thinking away from the previously widely held *unicellular* concept of immune recognition and function in which the prevailing thought had centered on the capacity of a single antigen-specific cell to recognize antigen and, upon so doing, to differentiate into a functionally mature effector cell mediating either humoral (antibody) immunity in the case of the bone marrow system or cell-mediated (delayed hypersensitivity, transplantation reactions) immunity in the case of the thymus system.

Very shortly after these observations were made, a series of observations, at times utilizing more refined systems, provided the groundwork for understanding that among the advantages of such multicellular involvement in a given immune response was the establishment of a framework for complex regulatory mechanisms capable of guiding each response in appropriate directions at any given time. By the early 1970s, therefore, it was clear that T lymphocytes exerted sophisticated regulatory effects on other lymphocytes of both classes and in this way dictated, in a sense, the quality and magnitude of most immune responses (reviewed in Ref. 7). It should be stated that we now know that T cell regulation of the immune system spans the entire spectrum from enhancement to suppression and involves complex cellular interactions between T cells and macrophages, T cells and T cells, and T cells and B cells; moreover, T cells participating in different regulatory functions or exerting effector roles in cell-mediated immunity are now known to belong to the distinct subclasses identifiable by their phenotypic expressions of distinct cell surface antigenic markers (for comprehensive discussions, see Refs. 8–11).

In terms of interactions between T and B lymphocytes in humoral immune responses, a considerable amount of information has been obtained in studies employing essentially 2 types of experimental models. The first type is a "physiologic" model system in the sense that it duplicates what presumably occurs between isogeneic cells in the intact individual. The second model is somewhat nonphysiologic in the sense that although the regulatory events appear to be identical to physiologic responses, the manner in which the model is established involves relatively artificial conditions. This latter model, which has been termed the "allogeneic effect," represents a phenomenon in which regulatory influences are exerted by allogeneic T cells interacting with histoincompatible T or B lymphocytes via cell surface histocompatibility antigens (reviewed in Ref. 12).

Examples of these 2 models are schematically illustrated in Figure 2. Inbred guinea pigs are immunized with a hapten-carrier conjugate of 2,4-dinitrophenyl –

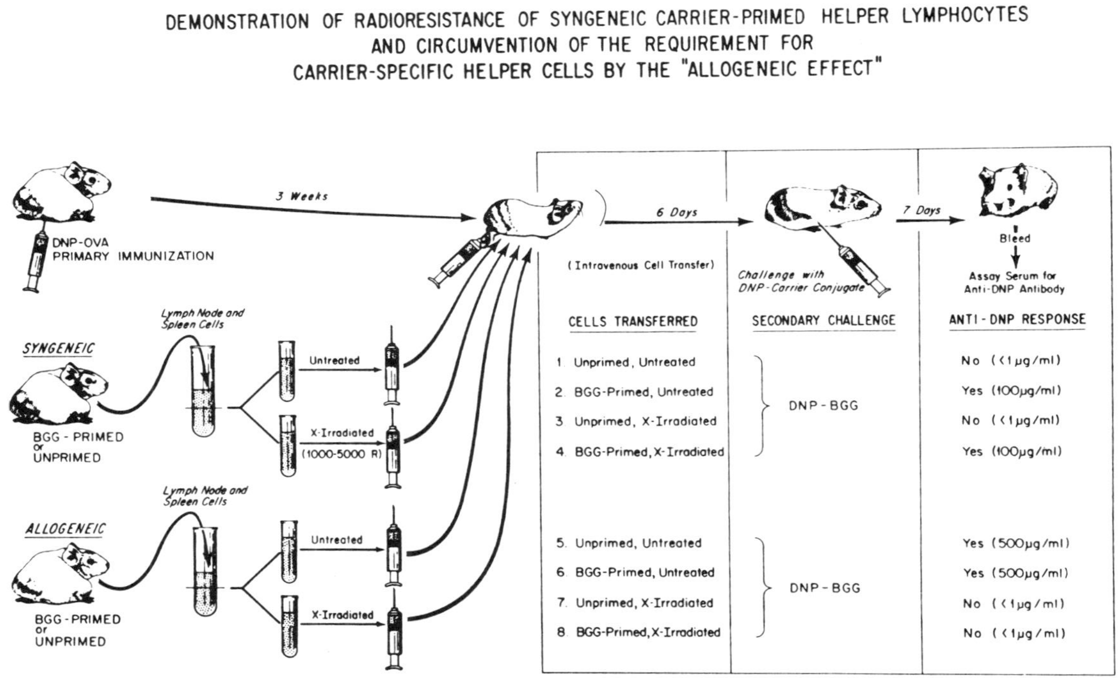

Fig. 2. Figs. 2, 4, and 5 reprinted from [23] with permission.

(DNP)-ovalbumin(OVA). Three weeks later, lymph node and spleen cells from syngeneic or allogeneic guinea pig donors are transferred intravenously into the DNP-OVA-primed recipients. The donors of lymphoid cells are either unprimed or previously primed to an unrelated carrier antigen such as bovine gamma globulin (BGG). The donor lymphoid cells are either transferred directly without treatment, or are subjected to x irradiation in vitro prior to cell transfer. Six days after cell transfer, the recipient guinea pigs are secondarily challenged with DNP-BGG and then bled 7 days later to measure the secondary anti-DNP antibody response. The first 4 groups (1–4) demonstrate the results obtained when syngeneic cells are transferred, while the latter 4 groups (5–8) illustrate the consequences of allogeneic cell transfers.

As shown here, unprimed syngeneic cells fail to provide a cooperative helper T-cell effect whether untreated or x-irradiated (groups 1 and 3). In contrast, syngeneic BGG-primed cells provide an excellent cooperative effect in permitting DNP-OVA-primed recipients to respond to DNP-BGG (group 2). This helper activity, known to be a reflection of T cell function in the BGG-primed population, is maintained even after exposure of these cells to x irradiation (group 4) indicating that little or no proliferation is required for such helper cells to function. The results obtained with allogeneic cells provide a striking contrast to those observed with the syngeneic cells. First, transfer of allogeneic lymphocytes results in a markedly greater helper activity which is demonstrable irrespective of whether or not such cells were obtained from donors specifically primed to the carrier, BGG (groups 5 and 6). Moreover, this allogeneic effect is completely abrogated if the donor cells are subjected to x irradiation prior to cell transfer (groups 7 and 8). Through a series of detailed studies, conclusive evidence was obtained that this allogeneic effect is a consequence of a transplantation reaction between the T lymphocytes of the donor population and the histoincompatible DNP-primed B lymphocytes of the host recipient (reviewed in Ref. 12).

After considerable analysis of the information obtained from studies with these 2 seemingly diverse model systems, it was found that the following remarkable parallels can be drawn between them insofar as their characteristic features: 1) The regulation by T cells is manifested on both T and B lymphocytes. 2) The net consequences of such regulation spans an entire spectrum of immunologic balance ranging from enhancement at one end to suppression at the other. 3) The initial cellular events occur at very definite surface membrane sites encoded by genes in the major histocompatibility complex.

It was the obvious importance of the third point above in the very potent regulatory influence exerted by the allogeneic effect, a phenomenon constituted by allogeneic cells interacting at histocompatible antigens on the cell surface, which suggested the possibility that such cell surface histocompatibility antigen molecules may, in fact, be intimately involved in cell-cell interactions occurring under physiologic conditions within an intact individual. This subject will be discussed more fully in the following sections.

GENETIC CONTROL OF IMMUNE RESPONSES

Another revolutionary series of concepts that have evolved during the past decade have been those concerned with the role of the major histocompatibility gene complex (MHC) in the immune system. For many years, gene products of the MHC (histocompatibility antigens) were studied in terms of their widely recognized function as major determinants of incompatibility in transplantation reactions. Extensive analyses have been made of the MHC in several species, and particularly the HLA system of humans (reviewed in Ref. 13) and the *H-2* system of mice (reviewed in Ref. 14). In the mid 1960s fundamental discoveries were made by Benacerraf and McDevitt and their respective co-workers that demonstrated for the first time a function of MHC genes in the control of immune responses to antigens other than those related in any obvious way to transplantation antigens and/or reactions (for reviews see Refs. 15, 16). The basic observations of these investigators were that individual strains of guinea pigs and mice differed in their capacities to develop immune responses to defined synthetic antigens. Responder strains and nonresponder strains were distinguished by their ability or inability to manifest both cell-mediated (delayed hypersensitivity) and humoral (antibody production) immune responses to the relevant antigens.

Studies utilizing congenic-resistant strains of mice which differed from one another only at the *H-2* gene complex established the linkage of responder or nonresponder status to genes in the MHC, and the MHC genes controlling such responses were termed immune response or *Ir* genes [15]. Such genes were shown to be inherited in mendelian fashion as autosomal dominant traits in most instances, although more recently the responder phenotype has been shown in selective cases to be expressed as a result of gene complementation, thus implicating the involvement of at least 2 *Ir* genes in the control of such responses (reviewed in Ref. 16). Analyses designed to locate the position of *Ir* genes in the MHC were conducted with recombinant strains of mice differing from one another by defined intra-*H-2* crossover events. These studies established the fact that *Ir* genes are distinct from the terminal *K* (left) or *D* (right) regions of the complex which had previously been shown to contain the genes encoding the major transplantation antigens detected most readily by serologic and tissue grafting techniques. Thus, *Ir* genes were found to reside in a new region, adjacent to and to the right of the *K* region, which was appropriately designated the *I* region [17]. A schematic illustration of the defined genetic regions and subregions of the mouse *H-2* complex as it is presently understood is shown in Figure 3.

In view of the facts that 1) all responses controlled by *Ir* genes involved the participation of T lymphocytes, 2) the specificity of such control appeared to be of a high order, and 3) the nature of the molecules functioning as antigen receptors on T cells was uncertain and initially appeared to be different from the

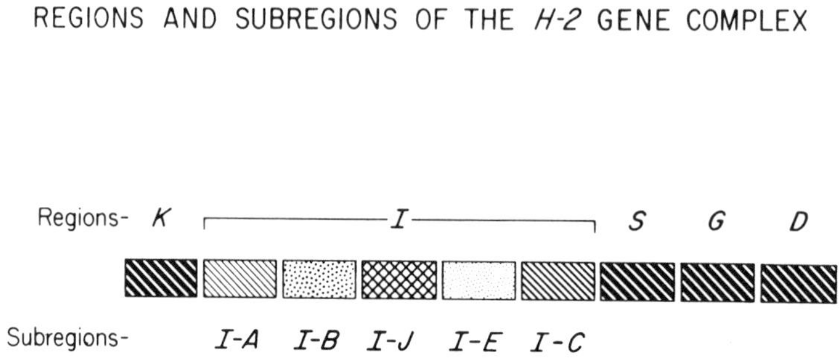

Fig. 3. Figs. 3 and 6 reprinted from [11] with permission.

Ig molecules serving as receptors on B lymphocytes, it was proposed several years ago that *Ir* genes encoded the molecular products functioning as T-cell receptors [15]. Indeed, this notion prompted considerable speculation and experimentation during the past 5 years and is still regarded by a few investigators as a valid possibility; however, the bulk of both direct and indirect evidence presently available tends to negate this possibility (see Ref. 11). Thus, it was established by studies performed initially by Ramseier and Lindenmann [18], and more recently by Binz and Wigzell [2] and Rajewsky et al [3] that T-cell receptors possess identical idiotypic determinants as found on Ig receptors on B cells. Since idiotypic determinants are characteristic of the region comprising the specific antigen-combining site, these findings strongly indicate that the variable (*V*) region genes encoding antigen specificity in immunoglobulins are also responsible for dictating specificity of T-cell receptors.

INVOLVEMENT OF MAJOR HISTOCOMPATIBILITY COMPLEX GENES IN CELL-CELL INTERACTIONS

As discussed above, studies on the phenomenon known as the allogeneic effect demonstrated that the final pathway of this phenomenon involved interactions at the histocompatibility molecules on the cell surface of the target T or B cells whose responses were being measured in the system. This fact led to the consideration that perhaps precisely the same pathway was involved in syngeneic interactions, occurring perhaps by similar molecular mechanisms. In order to test this possibility, a series of experiments was conducted to investigate whether physiologic T-B cell interactions in the mouse involved genetic restrictions associated with MHC genes. Such experiments were conducted utilizing a technique in which primed T and B lymphocytes were adoptively transferred to irradiated recipients under conditions specially designed to circumvent detectable nonspecific allogeneic effects. A schematic summary of the complex protocol employed in such experiments is illustrated in Figure 4 (see Ref. 19 for full description of the system).

The basic observation from such experiments was that antigen-specific T cells are capable of providing specific helper function for primed B cells of histocompatible, but *not* of histoincompatible, donor origin in secondary antibody responses of IgG class [19, 20]. Extensive genetic analyses were then conducted in attempts to define the location or locations of the genes controlling such interactions. In Figure 5 are compiled all of the results from studies which were designed to localize the gene(s) involved in controlling optimal T-B cell interactions. Such cell interaction or *CI* genes have been mapped within the *H-2* gene complex, and more specifically, to the *I-A* and/or *I-B* subregions, by utilizing mixtures of T and B lymphocytes from appropriate genetic recombinant inbred strains of mice with known identities and differences at various *H-2* regions and subregions (refer again to Figure 3).

In the middle panel of Figure 5 are shown the regions and subregions of the *H-2* complex. In various cell combinations studied, the presence of gene identities are shown by closed circles, whereas gene differences are indicated by open circles. The capacities of the various cell combinations to develop a cooperative response are shown in the far right panel. Fifteen cell combinations are shown, being numbered on the far left of the figure. The capacity to obtain responses in cell combinations 1 and 2, but not in 3 and 4, demonstrate that *CI* genes are, indeed, in the *H-2* complex since identities and differences at *H-2* determine the outcome of responses between such mixtures. Non-*H-2* or background genes are not involved, as evidenced by the capacity of cell combination 2 to give a positive response despite the existence of differences in background genes. This is further substantiated by the inability of cell combination 4 to cooperate where all background genes are identical, but differences exist in all *H-2* genes. The positive response in cell combination 5 reflects the capacity of reciprocal mixtures of parental and F_1 hybrid T and B cells to effectively interact in the system when conventional antigens are employed. (Exceptions to this finding occur when antigens controlled by *Ir* genes are utilized, as will be described below.) This is an important point since cell-cell interactions in parent-F_1 mixtures rule out the existence of: 1) Nonspecific blocking phenomena due to presence of foreign alloantigens (from the other parent) on the cell surface and 2) nonspecific suppression due to an allogeneic cell interaction.

The data from cell combinations 6–15 in Figure 5 illustrate the manner in which *CI* genes were mapped to the *I-A* and/or *I-B* subregions by these studies. This conclusion follows from the fact that in all combinations tested, effective cooperative interactions have been obtained whenever gene identities in *I-A* and/or *I-B* exist, and conversely, T and B cell mixtures that have differed in these 2 subregions have failed to display cooperative responses. The presence or

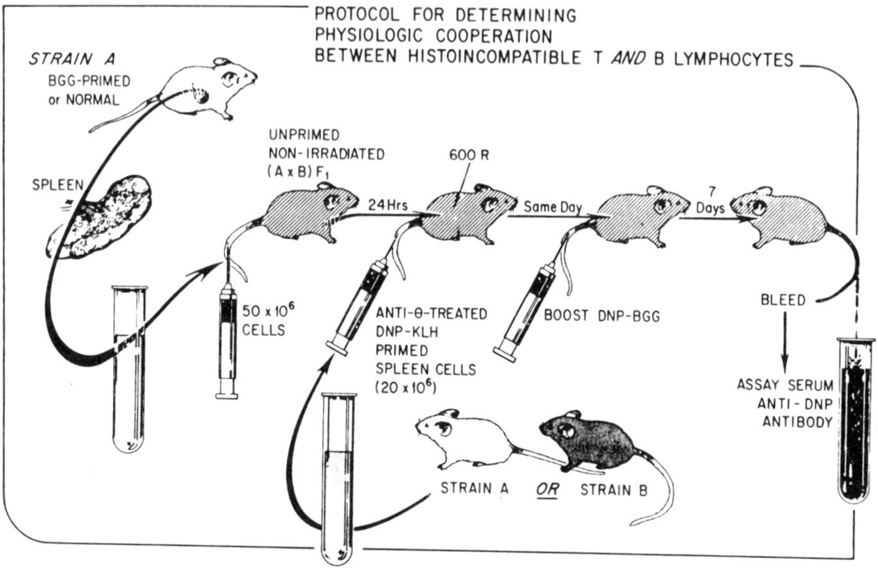

Fig. 4. Protocol for determining physiologic cooperation between histoincompatible T and B lymphocytes. Starting at the top left, spleen cells are obtained from carrier-primed mice (in this case, BGG) or normal mice of Strain A. These spleen cells are transferred intravenously into a nonirradiated, unprimed recipient which is an F_1 hybrid between Strain A and Strain B parents. Twenty-four hours later, this recipient, containing either carrier-primed or normal Strain A cells, is irradiated in a manner which abolishes graft-versus-host reactivity, but leaves intact the carrier-specific helper activity of the original primed donor inoculum. At this time, a second cell transfer is performed using spleen cells from either Strain A or Strain B donors previously immunized to DNP-KLH; these cells are first treated with anti-θ serum plus complement, a procedure which eliminates T lymphocytes. A second challenge is made with DNP-BGG and the mice are bled 7 days later for measurement of anti-DNP antibodies. In this manner, one can ascertain which combination or combinations of donor origin T and B lymphocytes can or cannot cooperatively interact to give secondary anti-DNP responses.

absence of gene identities in other regions or combinations of regions of *H-2*, such as *K, I-C, S, G,* or *D* does not appear to play a determining role.

The original interpretation of the collective observations mentioned above was that these genetic restrictions reflected the existence of cell surface molecules, distinct from antigen-specific receptors, that play a crucial role in mediating effective cell-cell interactions between T and B lymphocytes [19, 20]. These membrane components were assumed to be gene products of the *H-2* complex, and it was postulated that genetic identity between the T cell and the B cell was necessary for the relevant T-cell surface molecules to bind to the corresponding B-cell molecules, which were termed "acceptor" sites, for effective

MAPPING OF *CI* GENES CONTROLLING T-B CELL COOPERATIVE RESPONSES WITHIN THE *H-2* GENE COMPLEX

● GENE IDENTITIES ○ GENE DIFFERENCES

CELL COMBINATION	BACKGROUND GENOTYPE	*H-2* REGIONS AND SUB-REGIONS K	I: I-A	I: I-B	I: I-C	S	G	D	COOPERATIVE RESPONSE
1	●	●	●	●	●	●	●	●	YES
2	○	●	●	●	●	●	●	●	YES
3	○	○	○	○	○	○	○	○	NO
4	●	○	○	○	○	○	○	○	NO
5		●/○	●/○	●/○	●/○	●/○	●/○	●/○	YES
6		●	●	●	●	●	●	○	YES
7		●	●	●	●	○	○	○	YES
8		●	●	●	○	○	○	○	YES
9		●	●	●	○	○	○	●	YES
10		○	●	●	○	○	○	●	YES
11		○	●	●	●	●	●	●	YES
12		○	○	○	○	○	○	●	NO
13		○	○	○	●	●	●	●	NO
14		●	○	○	○	○	○	●	NO
15		●	○	○	○	○	○	○	NO

Fig. 5. Mapping of *CI* genes controlling T-B cell cooperative responses within the *H-2* gene complex.

interactions between primed T and B lymphocytes in development of antibody responses. Subsequently, the respective molecules were defined as cell interaction (CI) molecules and the *I* region genes coding them as *CI* genes [21].

A schematic illustration of how this concept is envisaged is illustrated in Figure 6. In this figure, cell interactions between allogeneic and syngeneic T and B lymphocytes are depicted. The flow on the left side illustrates the interaction between syngeneic T and B cells after or during antigen encounter by the respective cell types. Presumably, antigen activation of the T cell is facilitated by appropriate CI molecules on the surface of the macrophage or other suitable cell (not shown). Note that the interaction between syngeneic T and B cells (middle of diagram) is shown as occurring via the triangular CI molecules on the surfaces of both cells and that 2 alternative molecular mechanisms for this type of interaction are depicted: 1) Homologous or "like-like" interaction schematically indicated by alignment of the respective molecules and 2) complementary interaction depicted by the T cell molecule binding to the B cell CI site. The latter possibility has also been recently termed "dual recognition." The flow on the right side of Figure 6 illustrates the interaction between allogeneic T and B cells in which the histoincompatible T cell reacts at the same CI site on the B cell but in this case via an alloantigen-specific receptor. The B cell in both cases of syngeneic and allogeneic interactions goes on to the same consequence, namely, differentiation.

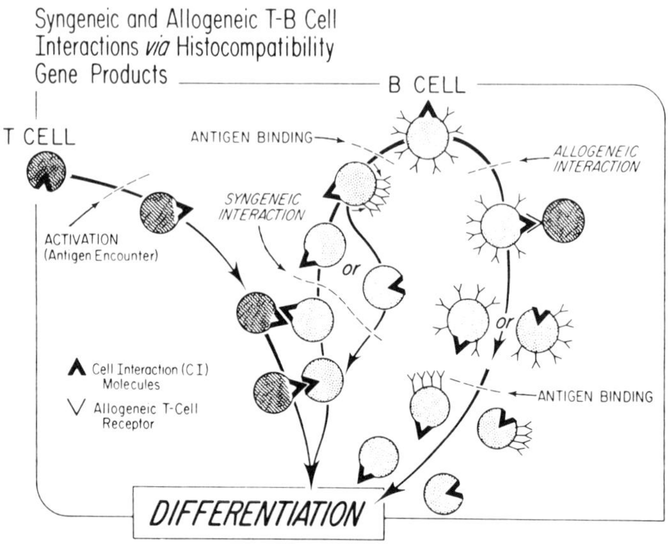

Fig. 6. Syngeneic and allogeneic T-B cell interactions *via* histocompatibility gene products

The point to be emphasized here is that the critical common feature of these 2 types of interactions is the molecular interaction occurring at the CI site on the B cell resulting in a requisite stimulus for further differentiation. This, in essence, is the predominant feature of the cell-interaction molecule concept. It is clearly not possible at the present time to make a valid conclusion as to whether interactions at the CI site(s) under physiologic circumstances occur by homology or complementarity, and distinguishing between these 2 possible molecular mechanisms for physiologic interactions will depend upon more precise biochemical analyses in the future. Nevertheless, it is germane to point out that the inferences of the 2 alternative mechanisms are substantial in that homologous interactions imply that the CI molecules on the respective cells are products of identical genes, whereas complementarity implies the reaction of a receptor entity on the T cell with a CI molecule on the target B cell (or T cell or macrophage), the respective molecules being products of distinct genes.

CONCLUDING REMARKS

In preceding sections of this paper, attention has been drawn to 2 major points that have become established in recent years in the field of basic immunobiology. The first point is that the immune system is regulated by a highly complex network of cell-cell interactions which are responsible for maintaining a finely-tuned balance of homeostasis assuring the well-being and integrity of the healthy individual. The second point is that it appears highly likely that such processes of cell-cell communication in the immune system are mediated through reactions occurring between cell surface molecules encoded by genes located in the major histocompatibility gene complex. The broad extension of the second point is that communication in the immune system occurs by a process of "self-recognition," a concept not really that revolutionary when one considers that self-recognition appears to be a fundamental biologic process concerned with the control of many types of developmental and differentiation events in both the plant and lower animal kingdoms. It may well be that similar processes of self-recognition are involved in the control of development and differentiation of other organ systems in complex multicellular organisms, and if such notions that have arisen as a consequence of analysis of the immune system pertain, one might well expect that the relevant molecules involved in such self-recognition events in other organ systems may also be gene products of the major histocompatibility gene complex. This, of course, is highly speculative and will require direct experimentation to prove or disprove its validity.

ACKNOWLEDGMENTS

I am grateful to all of my colleagues who participated in studies for our laboratory and to Ms. Judy Henneke for excellent secretarial assistance in the preparation of the manuscript.

Figure 1 reprinted from Katz DH: Genetic control of immune response: A dynamic interplay between genes, cells, and molecules. In Schmidtke JR, Ferguson RM (eds): "Immunology for the Practicing Physician." New York: Plenum Press, 1977, p 33 with permission. Figures 2, 4, and 5 reprinted from Katz DH: Interactions between T and B lymphocytes in immune responses. J Invest Dermatol 65:347, 1975 with permission. Figures 3 and 6 reprinted from Katz DH: "Lymphocyte Differentiation, Recognition and Regulation." New York: Academic Press, 1977 with permission.

REFERENCES

1. Unanue ER: The regulatory role of macrophages in antigenic stimulation. Adv Immunol 15:95, 1972.
2. Binz H, Wigzell H: Antigen-binding, idiotypic receptors from T lymphocytes. An analysis as to their biochemistry, genetics and use as immunogens to produce specific immune tolerance. Cold Spring Harbor Symp Quant Biol 41:275, 1977.

3. Rajewsky K, Hämmerling GJ, Black SJ, Berek C, Eichmann K: T lymphocyte receptor analysis by anti-idiotypic stimulation. In Katz DH, Benacerraf B (eds): "The Role of Products of the Histocompatibility Gene Complex in Immune Responses." New York: Academic Press, 1976, pp 445–453.
4. Claman HN, Chaperon EA, Triplett RF: Thymus-marrow cell combinations. Synergism in antibody production. Proc Soc Exp Biol Med 122:1167, 1966.
5. Davies AJS, Leuchars E, Wallis V, Marchant R, Elliott EV: The failure of thymus-derived cells to produce antibody. Transplantation 5:222, 1967.
6. Mitchell GF, Miller JFAP: Cell to cell interaction in the immune response. II. The source of hemolysin-forming cells in irradiated mice given bone marrow and thymus or thoracic duct lymphocytes. J Exp Med 128:821, 1968.
7. Katz DH, Benacerraf B: The regulatory influence of activated T cells on B cell responses to antigen. Adv Immunol 15:1, 1972.
8. Gershon RK: T cell control of antibody production. Contemp Top Immunol 3:1, 1973.
9. Cantor H, Weissman I: Development and function of subpopulations of thymocytes and T lymphocytes. Prog Allergy 20:1, 1976.
10. Cantor H, Boyse EA: Regulation of cellular and humoral immune responses by T cell subclasses. Cold Spring Harbor Symp Quant Biol 41:23, 1977.
11. Katz DH: "Lymphocyte Differentiation, Recognition, and Regulation." New York: Academic Press, 1977.
12. Katz DH: The allogeneic effect on immune responses. Model for regulatory influences of T lymphocytes on the immune system. Transplant Rev 12:141, 1972.
13. Bach FH, van Rood JJ: The major histocompatibility complex. N Engl J Med 295: 806–812, 872–878, 927–934, 1976.
14. Klein J: An attempt at an interpretation of the mouse H-2 complex. Contemp Top Immunobiol 5:297, 1976.
15. Benacerraf B, McDevitt HO: Histocompatibility-linked immune response genes. Science 175:273, 1972.
16. Benacerraf B, Katz DH: The nature and function of histocompatibility-linked immune response genes. In Benacerraf B (ed): "Immunogenetics and Immunodeficiency." London: Medical and Technical Publishing, 1975, pp 117–177.
17. McDevitt HO, Deak BD, Shreffler DC, Klein J, Stimpling JH, Snell GD: Genetic control of the immune response. Mapping of the *Ir-1* locus. J Exp Med 135:1259, 1972.
18. Ramseier H, Lindenmann J: Aliotypic antibodies. Transplant Rev 10:57, 1972.
19. Katz DH, Hamaoka T, Benacerraf B: Cell interactions between histoincompatible T and B lymphocytes. II. Failure of physiologic cooperative interactions between T and B lymphocytes from allogeneic donor strains in humoral response to hapten-protein conjugates. J Exp Med 137:1405, 1973.
20. Katz DH, Hamaoka T, Dorf ME, Benacerraf B: Cell interactions between histoincompatible T and B lymphocytes. III. Demonstration that the H-2 gene complex determines successful physiologic lymphocyte interactions. Proc Natl Acad Sci USA 70: 2626, 1973.
21. Katz DH, Benacerraf B: The function and interrelationships of T cell receptors, Ir genes and other histocompatibility gene products. Transplant Rev 22:175, 1975.
22. Katz DH: Genetic control of immune response: A dynamic interplay between genes, cells, and molecules. In Schmidtke JR, Ferguson RM (eds): "Immunology for the Practicing Physician." New York: Plenum Press, 1977, p 33.
23. Katz DH: Interactions between T and B lymphocytes in immune responses. J Invest Dermatol 65:347, 1975.

Adenosine Deaminase (ADA) and Other Enzyme Abnormalities in Immune Deficiency States*

Randall M. Goldblum, MD, Frank C. Schmalstieg, MD, PhD, J. Arly Nelson, PhD, and Gordon C. Mills, PhD

INTRODUCTION

New pathways of investigation into the metabolic requirements of immune function were opened by Giblett et al [1] in 1972, when two patients with severe deficiencies of T lymphocytes were found to be deficient in an enzyme involved in purine metabolism. The deficiency of erythrocyte adenosine deaminase (ADA) was quickly confirmed in other patients deficient in T and B cells, who exhibited immunologic findings consistent with severe combined immunodeficiency disease [2–4]. Despite low enzyme activity in all tissues of ADA-deficient children [5], the major clinical findings have been limited to the immunologic abnormalities and a mild bone dysplasia.

A causal relationship was postulated between this abnormality of purine metabolism and immunodeficiency since population studies had failed to demonstrate normal individuals with ADA deficiency and since all individuals severely deficient in the enzyme were immunologically impaired [6]. Heterozygous carriers of this autosomal recessive defect were found to have half-normal enzyme activity but no impairment of the immunologic system [1]. Furthermore, a critical level of ADA activity for immunologic function was suggested by the finding that individuals with an allotypic variant of the enzyme having approximately 10% of normal catalytic activity are immunologically normal [7].

*This work was supported in part by a grant from The National Institutes of Health, grant DHEW RR-00073-14, General Clinical Research Centers Branch, Division of Research Facilities and Resources; and by grant #6-130 from The National Foundation–March of Dimes.

Birth Defects: Original Article Series, Volume XIV, Number 6A, pages 73–84

Further evidence for the importance of the purine catabolic and scavenger pathway was provided by Giblett's demonstration of purine nucleoside phosphorylase (NP) deficiency in a child with T-lymphocyte deficiency [8]. This finding, now confirmed in six other cases [9–11], may also provide an opportunity to find the metabolic aberration, common to two enzyme deficiences, which may mediate the T-lymphocyte dysfunction.

Diminished activity of two other enzymes in purine metabolism, 5′-nucleotidase [12] and hypoxanthine-guanine phosphoribosyl transferase [13] has been reported in association with diminished B-lymphocyte number and function. However, since these associations have not been confirmed, we will focus our discussion on ADA and NP deficiencies.

PURINE METABOLISM

The major pathways of purine metabolism in humans are shown in Figure 1A. The relative activities of ADA and adenosine kinase (adenosine→adenosine monophosphate) are important in determining the amount of adenosine which contributes to the formation of adenine nucleotides or that is ultimately catabolized to uric acid. While NP is important in this same pathway, it may also regulate the levels of guanosine and deoxyguanosine. Figure 1B outlines the sources of intracellular nucleotides from de novo synthesis and salvage of adenine, hypoxanthine, and guanine. Both processes require phosphoribosyl pyrophosphate (PP-ribose-P). Two mechanisms which regulate purine and pyrimidine metabolism and may be of importance in ADA and NP deficiency are shown in Figure 2. The intracellular level of PP-ribose-P modulates the rate of purine biosynthesis and is itself controlled by a complex balance between synthesis and utilization (Fig. 2A). For instance, in the absence of hypoxanthine-guanine phosphoribosyl transferase or hypoxanthine production, PP-ribose-P may accumulate and lead to increased purine synthesis. Figure 2B depicts the mechanisms by which adenosine may lead to increased levels of cAMP by increasing substrate adenosine triphosphate (ATP) and activating adenyl cyclase [14].

IN VITRO MODELS OF ADA AND NP DEFICIENCY

While the toxicity of adenosine for cultured cells has long been appreciated, interest in the effect of adenosine on lymphocytes was enhanced by the discovery of hereditary ADA deficiency. Table 1 summarizes studies of the inhibitory activity of adenosine on lymphocyte cultures. As expected, the inhibitory dose is lower in cultures simultaneously treated with ADA inhibitors. A concentration of 5–50 μM causes a 50% inhibition (ID_{50}) of the measured lymphocyte activity [15, 16]. In addition to the effects on cell division, Green and Chan [17] demonstrated diminished intracellular pyrimidines in adenosine-treated lymphoid

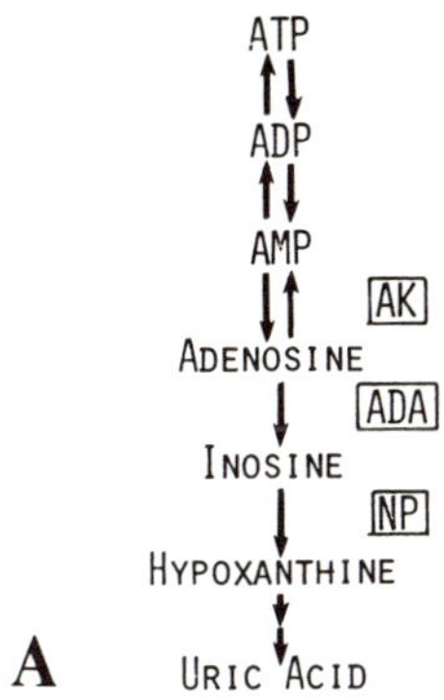

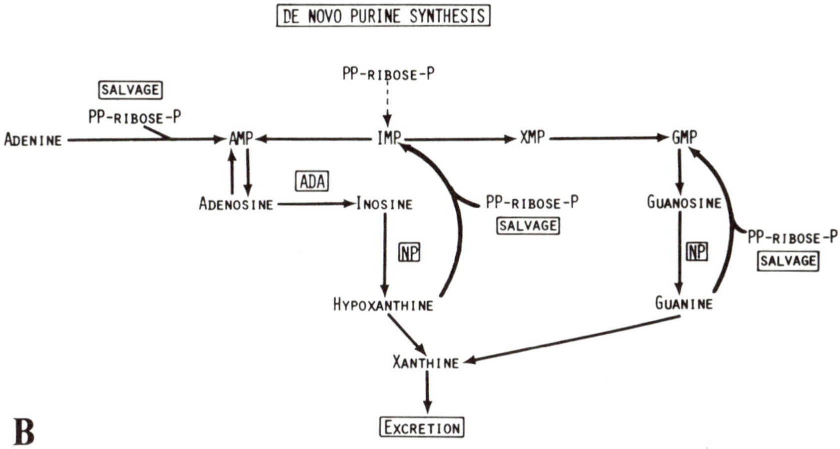

Fig. 1. Pathways of purine metabolism. A) Interconversion and catabolism of adenine nucleotides. ADA, Adenosine deaminase; NP, purine nucleoside phosphorylase; AK, adenosine kinase. B) Synthesis, salvage, and excretion of purines. Ac, Adenyl cyclase.

cell lines. This effect was possibly due to the reduction of the PP-ribose-P level by increased adenine nucleotides. Wolberg et al [18] did not confirm that finding in murine splenic lymphocytes, but they did find that adenosine caused a rise in the level of cAMP, which correlated with inhibition of cell-mediated cytotoxicity.

These studies led to two major hypotheses for the effect of ADA deficiency on lymphoid cell division and function. However, despite further reports, it has not demonstrated conclusively that pyrimidine starvation or increased levels of cAMP are responsible for lymphocyte dysfunction in adenosine-treated cells.

The in vitro toxicities of inosine and guanosine, two substrates of NP, have not been examined extensively. In one study using mouse lymphosarcoma cells [19], inosine (up to 2 mM) did not inhibit growth, while the combination of adenosine

TABLE 1. Adenosine Toxicity in Lymphocyte Cultures

Investigator, reference	Lymphocyte source	ADA inhibitor	Effective adenosine concentration (ID_{50}) (μM)
Hirschhorn et al [5]	Human blood	–	100
Green and Chan [17]	Lymphoid cell lines	–	1–3 (20 → ↓ pyrimidine)
Wolberg et al [18]	Mouse spleen	EHNA (7.9 μM)	
		–	150
		+	4.7
Carsen and Seegmiller [15]	Human blood	EHNA (50 μM)	
		–	500
		+	50 (DNA) 5 (protein)
Hovi et al [16]	Human blood	Corformycin (0.1 μM)	
		–	50
		+	10

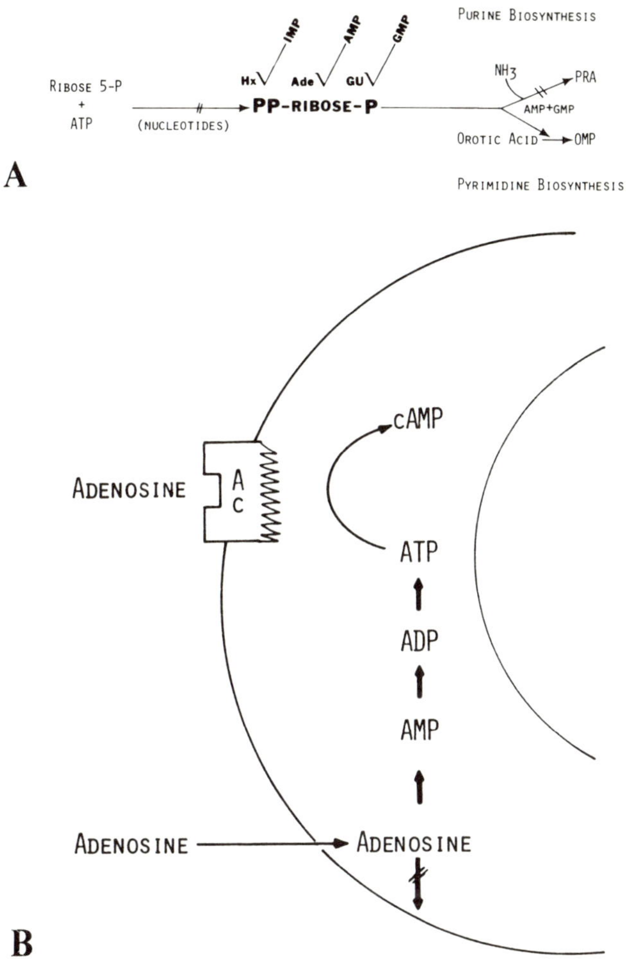

Fig. 2. A) The role of phosphoribosyl pyrophosphate (PP-ribose-P) in regulation of purine and pyrimidine biosynthesis. HX, Hypoxanthine; Ade, adenine; Gu, guanine; PRA, phosphoribosylanine; —//→, inhibition of reaction. B) The effect of adenosine on intracellular cAMP level. Ac, Membrane-bound adenyl cyclase.

(50 μM) and inosine (20 μM) was inhibitory. Large concentrations of guanosine (2 mM) have recently been demonstrated to inhibit [^{3}H]-thymidine incorporation by phytohemagglutinin (PHA)-stimulated human lymphocytes [20]. Unfortunately, these studies are hampered by the lack of a potent NP inhibitor.

The effect of exogenous deoxyribonucleosides on DNA synthesis in PHA-stimulated human lymphocytes has also been examined by Tattersall et al [21].

Interestingly, both deoxyadenosine and deoxyguanosine inhibit [^{3}H]-thymidine incorporation, probably by reducing deoxyribonucleotide triphosphate levels.

PURINE INTERMEDIATES IN ENZYME DEFICIENCY PATIENTS

The effect of ADA deficiency on the levels of purine intermediates in the cell and biologic fluids has been studied in only a few patients with this disorder. One patient, now almost 3 years old, was found to have severe combined immunodeficiency and ADA deficiency when he was evaluated for recurrent and chronic infections at the age of 2 months. In the absence of a compatible bone marrow donor, the patient was maintained in a clean but nonsterile environment, and extensive studies of purine and pyrimidine metabolism were carried out [22, 23].

No evidence of pyrimidine starvation was found. The results of the purine studies are summarized in Figure 3. Adenosine was increased (0.7–3 μM) in plasma but not in urine. Adenine nucleotides, especially ATP, were moderately increased in erythrocytes, but were dramatically increased in lymphocytes, as was cAMP. The urine contained large amounts of both adenine and deoxyadenosine. While at least part of the adenine appears to be derived during analysis from deoxyadenosine [24], it is clear that adenine was present in the urine and erythrocytes in concentrations far greater than normal. The source of this compound has not been determined. No evidence for pyrimidine depletion of erythrocytes or lymphocytes or for orotic aciduria was found. The high levels of

	PLASMA	URINE	RBC	LYMPHOCYTES
Adenosine	↑	→	→	→
AMP			→	
ADP			→	↑
ATP			↑	↑↑
cAMP				↑
Deoxyadenosine	*	↑	→	↑
Adenine	↑*	↑*	↑↑	↑
Pyrimidines			→	↑

Fig. 3. Purine and pyrimidine abnormalities in an ADA-deficient patient. ↑ One upward arrow, increased concentration; ↑ ↑ two upward arrows, greatly increased concentration; → sideways arrow, normal concentration. An asterisk indicates that a portion of the adenine found was produced by acid hydrolysis of deoxyadenosine during the assay procedures.

lymphocyte ATP and plasma adenosine have been confirmed in one other ADA-deficient patient [25].

The levels of purine intermediates in serum or urine of four patients with NP deficiency have been reported [9, 26]. The NP substrates, inosine and guanosine, were both markedly elevated (13–99 μM and 5.6–29 μM, respectively) in the serum. The urine contained large amounts of these ribonucleosides and, interestingly, deoxyguanosine and deoxyinosine were also demonstrated. Plasma adenosine was not detected, but the sensitivity of the methods used may not have been adequate to measure moderately increased levels of adenosine. As expected, hypoxanthine and uric acid were decreased in the urine. However, total purine excretion was markedly increased, as was erythrocyte PP-ribose-P in one case [26]. These findings are consistent with the importance of hypoxanthine and hypoxanthine-guanine phosphoribosyl transferase in the utilization of PP-ribose-P and thereby control of de novo purine biosynthesis. Further comparison between the biochemical finding of ADA and NP deficiency has been hampered by the lack of intracellular nucleotide determinations in NP-deficient patients.

EFFECT OF ENZYME REPLACEMENT

Because the micromolar concentrations of adenosine which inhibit in vitro lymphocyte function are present in the plasma of ADA-deficient patients, it seemed likely that removal of adenosine might improve the immunologic functions of these patients. This hypothesis was first tested by Polmar and his colleagues by adding ADA to cultured blood lymphocytes from a patient with ADA deficiency [27]. A marked enhancement in the concanavalin A-induced proliferation of the lymphocytes was noted in his patient [27], while a moderate improvement was confirmed in ours [23]. In neither case, nor in one studied by Parkman et al [28], was uridine effective in enhancing the in vitro proliferative responses. In our patient, overnight incubation of lymphocytes with ADA led to a modest (25%) decrease in cAMP levels, an effect not noted on normal lymphocytes [22]. Similar studies on NP-deficient lymphocytes have not been reported.

The results of these in vitro studies in ADA deficiency encouraged Polmar and his co-workers [25] and our group [24] to pursue in vivo enzyme replacement using infusions of ADA-containing erythrocytes and plasma. Using special precautions to prevent the transfer of viable lymphocytes, both groups have tested this therapy for more than 17 months. The effect on the immune system of these and two other patients tested for a shorter period are summarized in Table II. In Polmar s case, the ADA endogenous activity in the lymphocytes was 6% of normal, and the lymphocyte number and proliferative response returned to normal in that patient within 10 and 3 days, respectively, following transfusion.

These changes were accompanied by a persistent decrease (though not to normal levels) of lymphocyte ATP.

The effects of red blood cell transfusion in our patient whose ADA levels were less than 1% of normal were much less marked. While statistically significant changes in the same immunologic parameters were noted in our patient, the changes were small (approximately twofold) and transient. The effect of transfusion waned, while 70% of the transfused erythrocyte ADA remained. The limited nature of the in vitro and in vivo reconstitution of immune function in our patient suggested either a loss of responsive lymphoid cells or inadequate biochemical correction. Sequential examination of the levels of purine intermediates after erythrocyte infusions (Fig. 4) favors the latter possibility. Both erythrocyte and lymphocyte ATP levels began to fall 4 days after infusion but quickly rose to preinfusion levels starting on day 8. The transient increases in lymphocyte number and proliferative responses to mitogen occurred approximately 10 and 13 days after infusion. Thus, it appears that despite infusion of large numbers of ADA-containing erythrocytes, we were unable to cause a persistent decrease in adenine nucleotides or immune reconstitution. Although too few patients have been treated by this modality, there appears to be a relationship between the residual ADA activity of lymphocytes and the outcome of ADA replacement therapy (Table 2).

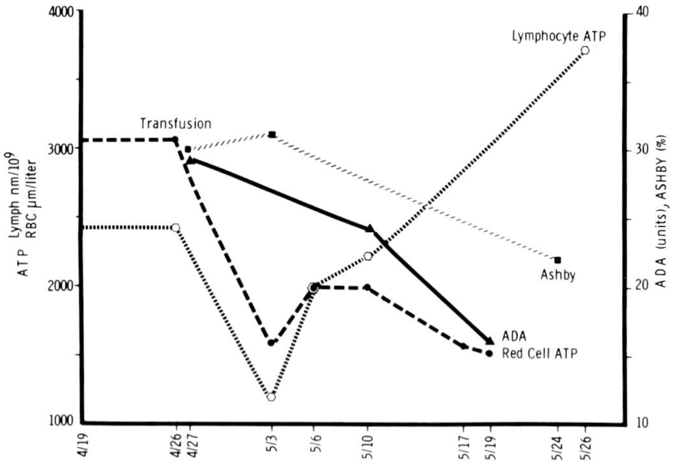

Fig. 4. The effect of red blood cell transfusion on erythrocyte ADA and ATP and lymphocyte ATP. The percentage of donor cells remaining in the patient's blood is indicated by the Ashby results. RBC, Red blood cells.

TABLE 2. Response to Red Blood Cells and Plasma Infusion in ADA Deficiency

Investigator, reference	Lymph ADA (%)	Increased lymphocytes	Increased T cells	Increased mitogen response	DHS	Increased immuno-globulins	Antibody formation
Polmar et al [25]	6	+	+	+	–	+	+
Schmalstieg et al [24]	< 1	±	±	±	–	+	–
Wolf et al [30][1]	10	+	+	Normal before	+	Normal before	Normal before
Ziegler (personal communication) (Sydney, Australia)	UD	–	–	–	?	±	?

[1]This patient was treated simultaneously with calf thymic peptides (thymosin).
DHS = Delayed hypersensitivity.

CONCLUSIONS

A deficiency of ADA or NP, two enzymes in the purine metabolic pathways, causes rather specific abnormalities in the development and function of T lymphocytes. Deficiency of ADA may also affect B lymphocytes, but this effect may be secondary to an inability of T lymphocytes to augment B-lymphocyte function. In vitro experiments suggest a role of purine nucleosides in the immunologic dysfunction and indicate several possible biochemical mechanisms.

Accumulation of the expected nucleosides has been demonstrated in the plasma of ADA- and NP-deficient subjects. Adenine nucleotides, including cAMP, have been found in increased amounts in the lymphocytes of ADA-deficient patients. Immunologic reconstitution after ADA replacement seems to correlate with the fall in lymphocyte ATP being either persistent [25] or transient [24]. However, whether adenine nucleotides are actually inhibitory to immune function is unproven.

A possible clue to the importance of the biochemical abnormalities demonstrated in ADA deficiency might come from comparative studies of NP-deficient patients. Inosine, demonstrated in the urine, plasma, and erythrocytes of these patients, is a weak inhibitor of ADA (K_i = 116 μM) [29]. Since the levels of inosine found in NP deficiency are below the K_i, this inhibition would not appear to be important. However, partial inhibition of ADA might lead to accumulation of adenine nucleotides in the presence of purine overproduction. Further studies of NP-deficient patients will be critical in this respect. Alternatively, guanosine nucleotides, also affected by NP deficiency, may have a direct effect on immunologic function. The role of deoxyribonucleosides demonstrated in both types of patients is at present unknown.

It seems clear that during the 5 years following Giblett's original description of ADA deficiency, important information concerning specific relationships between purine metabolism and immune function has begun to accumulate. Further understanding of this relationship should provide valuable information concerning the metabolic requirement for normal development and function of the immune system.

ACKNOWLEDGMENTS

The authors wish to express their appreciation to Ms. Betzy J. Finger for her secretarial and technical graphic assistance in the preparation of this manuscript, Dr. Linda T. May and Dr. James T. Howell for their assistance in the preparation of this manuscript, and the professional staff of the Clinical Research Center for their excellent patient care.

Dr. Schmalstieg is the recipient of a James W. McLaughlin Postdoctoral Fellowship, University of Texas Medical Branch, Galveston.

REFERENCES

1. Giblett ER, Anderson JE, Cohen F, Pollara B, Meuwissen HJ: Adenosine-deaminase deficiency in two patients with severely impaired cellular immunity. Lancet 2:1067–1069, 1972.
2. Dissing J, Knudsen B: Adenosine-deaminase deficiency and combined immunodeficiency syndrome. Lancet 2:1316, 1972.
3. Ochs HD, Yount JE, Giblett ER, Chen S-H, Scott CR, Wedgwood RJ: Adenosine-deaminase deficiency and severe combined immunodeficiency syndrome. Lancet 2: 1393–1394, 1973.
4. Yount J, Nichols P, Ochs HD, Hammar SP, Scott CR, Chen S-H, Giblett ER, Wedgwood RJ: Absence of erythrocyte adenosine deaminase associated with severe combined immunodeficiency. J Pediatr 84:173–177, 1974.
5. Hirschhorn R, Levytska V, Pollara B, Meuwissen HJ: Evidence for control of several different tissue-specific lysozymes of adenosine deaminase by a single genetic locus. Nature (New Biol) 246:200–202, 1973.
6. Meuwissen HJ, Pickering RJ, Moore EC, Pollara B: Impairment of adenosine deaminase activity in combined immunological deficiency disease. In Meuwissen HJ, Pickering RJ, Pollar B, Porter IH (eds): "Combined Immunodeficiency Disease and Adenosine Deaminase Deficiency." New York: Academic Press, 1975.
7. Jenkins T, Rabson AR, Nurse GT, Lane AB, Hopkinson DA: Deficiency of adenosine deaminase not associated with severe combined immunodeficiency. J Pediatr 89:732–736, 1976.
8. Giblett ER, Ammann AJ, Sandman R, Wara DW, Diamond LK: Nucleoside-phosphorylase deficiency in a child with severely defective T-cell immunity and normal B-cell immunity. Lancet 1:1010–1013, 1975.
9. Stoop JW, Zegers BJM, Hendrickx GFM, Siegenbeek van Heukelom LH, Staal GEJ, de Bree PK, Wadman SK, Ballieux RE: Purine nucleoside phosphorylase deficiency associated with selective cellular immunodeficiency. N Engl J Med 296:651–655, 1977.
10. Griscelli G, Hauret M, Ballet JJ: Inosine phosphorylase deficiency with fatal vaccinia gangrenosa. Presented at the Third Workshop International Cooperative Group for Bone Marrow Transplantation in Man, New York, August, 1976.
11. Biggar WD, Ozere RL: A variant form of nucleoside phosphorylase deficiency in two brothers with defective T-cell function. J Pediatr (in press).
12. Johnson SM, Asherson GL, Watts RWE, North ME, Allsop J, Webster ADB: Lymphocyte purine 5′-nucleotidase deficiency in primary hypogammaglobulinaemia. Lancet 1:168–170, 1977.
13. Allison AC, Watts RWE, Hovi T, Webster ADB: Immunological observations on patients with Lesch-Nyhan syndrome, and on the role of de-novo purine synthesis in lymphocyte transformation. Lancet 2:1179–1183, 1975.
14. Clark RB, Gross R, Su YF: Regulation of adenosine 3′:5′-monophosphate content in human astrocytoma cells by adenosine and adenine nucleotides. J Biol Chem 249:5296–5303, 1974.
15. Carson DA, Seegmiller JE: Effect of adenosine deaminase inhibition upon human lymphocyte blastogenesis. J Clin Invest 57:274–282, 1976.
16. Hovi T, Smyth JF, Allison AC: Role of adenosine deaminase in lymphocyte proliferation. Clin Exp Immunol 23:395–403, 1976.
17. Green H, Chan T-S: Pyrimidine starvation induced by adenosine in fibroblasts and lymphoid cells: Role of adenosine deaminase. Science 182:836–837, 1973.

18. Wolberg G, Zimmerman TP, Hiemstra K, Winston M, Chu LC: Adenosine inhibition of lymphocyte mediated cytolysis: Possible role of cyclic adenosine monophosphate. Science 187:957–959, 1975.
19. Ullman B, Cohen A, Martin DW Jr: Characterization of a cell culture model for the study of adenosine deaminase- and purine nucleoside phosphorylase-deficient immunologic disease. Cell 9:205–211, 1976.
20. Ochs U, Osborne W, Chen S-H, Scott CR: Human lymphocyte transformation following inhibition of purine nucleoside phosphorylase. Pediatr Res 11:491a, 1977.
21. Tattersall MHN, Ganeshaguru K, Hoffbrand AV: The effect of external deoxyribonucleosides on deoxyribonucleoside triphosphate concentrations in human lymphocytes. Bioche Pharmacol 24:1495–1498, 1975.
22. Mills GC, Schmalstieg FC, Trimmer KB, Goldman AS, Goldblum RM: Purine metabolism in adenosine deaminase deficiency. Proc Natl Acad Sci USA 73:2867–2871, 1976.
23. Schmalstieg FC, Nelson JA, Mills GC, Monahan TM, Goldman AS, Goldblum RM: Increased purine nucleotides in adenosine deaminase deficient lymphocytes. J Pediatr 91:48–51, 1977.
24. Schmalstieg FC, Mills GC, Nelson JA, May LT, Goldman AS, Goldblum RM: Limited effect of erythrocyte and plasma infusion in adenosine deaminase deficiency. Submitted for publication.
25. Polmar SH, Stern RC, Schwartz AL, Wetzler EM, Chase PA, Hirschhorn R: Enzyme replacement therapy for adenosine deaminase deficiency and severe combined immunodeficiency. N Engl J Med 295:1337–1343, 1976.
26. Cohen A, Doyle D, Martin DW Jr, Ammann AJ: Abnormal purine metabolism and purine overproduction in a patient deficient in purine nucleoside phosphorylase. N Engl J Med 295:1449–1454, 1976.
27. Polmar SH, Wetzler EM, Stern RC, Hirschhorn R: Restoration of in-vitro lymphocyte responses with exogenous adenosine deaminase in a patient with severe combined immunodeficiency. Lancet 2:743–746, 1975.
28. Parkman R, Gelfand EW, Rosen FS, Sanderson A, Hirschhorn R: Severe combined immunodeficiency and adenosine deaminase deficiency. N Engl J Med 292:714–719, 1975.
29. Agarwal RP, Sagar SM, Parks RE Jr: Adenosine deaminase from human erythrocytes: Purification and effects of adenosine analogs. Biochem Pharmacol 24:693–701, 1975.
30. Wolf J, Reid R, Anderson J, Rebuck J, Lightbody J, Johnson R, Uberti J, Weiss L: Cellular immunodeficiency (Nezelof) associated with ADA deficiency: Treatment with with thymosin and ADA enzyme replacement. J Reticuloendothel Soc 20:94a, 1976.

Malignancy in Children With and Without Genetically-Determined Immunodeficiencies

Beatrice D. Spector, BA, Guy S. Perry, III, BA, Kazimiera J. Gajl-Peczalska, MD, PhD, Peter Coccia, MD, Mark E. Nesbit, MD, and John H. Kersey, MD

The purpose of this report is to present data comparing the occurrence of childhood malignancies, particularly non-Hodgkin lymphoproliferative tumors, in 2 groups of patients. The 1st group consists of those children with genetically determined immunodeficiency diseases (GDID) who have developed malignancies in the course of their primary disease. Information about them comes from data collected for the Immunodeficiency-Cancer Registry located at the University of Minnesota [1]. The 2nd group of patients consists of children who have developed malignancy without prior immunodeficiency disease. Information about this group comes from 2 sources: 1) published reports by the National Cancer Institute's Third National Cancer Survey of newly diagnosed childhood malignancies occurring during the period 1969–1971; 2) data from a study of 79 children with newly diagnosed non-Hodgkin lymphomas or acute lymphocytic leukemia who were seen at the Pediatric Oncology Clinic at the University of Minnesota Hospitals [2, 3].

Before the description of the results of our comparison studies, attention should be called to *genetically determined* examples of immunodeficiencies of childhood associated with malignancy (Table 1). Table 1 lists the 11 diseases, variously named, in which have occurred reports of malignancy in patients with the disease. The diseases have in common laboratory-verified abnormalities of the B-lymphocyte system, abnormalities of the T-lymphocyte system, and, in several diseases, defects of both B-lymphocyte and T-lymphocyte function. For convenience, each of the 11 diseases is listed by the primary cell defect(s) identified for that disease. There are 5 diseases in the registry which are identified as combined B- and T-cell defects, 4 diseases which present as isolated B-cell immunodeficiencies, and 2 diseases recognized as primary T-cell immunodeficiencies. The inheritance pattern, where known, is included for each disorder [4–6].

Birth Defects: Original Article Series, Volume XIV, Number 6A, pages 85–89

TABLE 1. Genetically Determined Immunodeficiency Diseases (GDID) of Childhood Associated With Malignancy

Cellular defect	Inheritance pattern
Combined B- and T-cell defects:	
Severe combined immunodeficiency disease	X-linked, autosomal-recessive
Immunodeficiency with ataxia-telangiectasia	Autosomal-recessive
Immunodeficiency with thrombocytopenia and eczema (Wiskott-Aldrich syndrome)	X-linked
Immunodeficiency with normal or elevated serum gamma globulins	X-linked, variable[a]
Variable immunodeficiency – Childhood onset	Variable
B-Cell defects only:	
X-linked (Bruton) Agammaglobulinemia	X-linked
X-linked immunodeficiency with hyper IgM	X-linked
Selective IgA deficiency	Variable
Selective IgM deficiency	Variable
T-Cell defects only:	
Thymic hypoplasia (Di George syndrome)	Variable
Episodic lymphopenia and lymphocytotoxin	Variable

[a]Various modes of inheritance have been reported; also, possible multifactorial or unknown genetic bases, or no known genetic bases.

The first comparison to be made concerns the incidence of malignancies of various types reported in children with and without these genetic diseases involving the immune system. There are 154 children with one of these 11 diseases who are known to the registry to have developed a malignancy. In Table 2 are the results of the percent distribution of reported malignancies by histologic type, compared with "unselected" children, ie those children whose tumors were diagnosed during the Third National Cancer Survey. Young and Miller [2] analyzed these data and determined the 7 most common tumors of childhood; these 7 tumor types, listed in rank order in the unselected column include the following: leukemias (33.8%), central nervous system tumors (19.2%), lymphomas (10.6%) (6.2% non-Hodgkin lymphomas), neuroblastomas (6.4%), Wilms tumors (6.1%), bone tumors (4.5%), and rhabdomyosarcomata (3.6%). In contrast, children with GDID predominantly developed lymphomas (41.0% non-Hodgkin); leukemias were 2nd in frequency at 21.5% of the total. Except for a few central nervous system tumors, children with GDID did *not* develop other common childhood malignancies, although total numbers are small.

We now turn to an analysis of non-Hodgkin lymphoproliferative malignancies in children with and without laboratory documented genetically determined immunodeficiencies. Analyses of malignant lymphoid blast cells are routinely done on newly diagnosed non-Hodgkin lymphomas and lymphoid leukemias.

Kersey et al [3] have performed such analyses on 79 children at the University of Minnesota Hospitals and developed classification criteria which have been adopted for this report. These classification criteria of non-Hodgkin lymphomas and lymphoid leukemias into lymphocyte phenotypes are listed in Table 3. A malignancy is considered B-like in phenotype if > 70% of the malignant blast cells are surface immunoglobulin (SIg) positive and/or if the tumor has been diagnosed as a Burkitt lymphoma or a plasmacytoma, or has presented as an abdominal mass lesion. A malignancy is considered T-like in phenotype if malignant blast cells are E-rosette positive (in some cases HTLA positive as well as, or instead of, E-rosette positive) and/or the tumor presented as an anterior mediastinal (thymic) mass lesion. If neither B-like nor T-like markers were observed on malignant blast cells and if the tumor presented with bone marrow involvement *without* masses, it was labeled a "null" cell type. Table 4 displays the results of our analysis of non-Hodgkin lymphomas and lymphoid leukemias

TABLE 2. Incidence of Malignancy of Various Types in Children Under 15 Years of Age

Tumor type	Unselected children[a] (%)	Children with GDID[b] (%)	
Leukemia (all types)	33.8	21.5	(33)
Central nervous system	19.2	6.6	(10)
Lymphoma (all types)	10.6	63.0	(97)
Neuroblastoma	6.4	0.6	(1)
Wilms tumor	6.1	0.6	(1)
Bone tumors (all types)	4.5	0.0	(0)
Rhabdomyosarcoma	3.6	0.0	(0)
Other	15.8	7.8	(12)
Totals	100.0	100.0	(154)

[a]See [2, p 254].
[b]From Immunodeficiency-Cancer Registry; number of patients in parentheses.

TABLE 3. Classification Criteria of Non-Hodgkin Lymphomas and Leukemias Into Lymphocyte Phenotypes

Classification criteria	Lymphocyte phenotype
Surface immunoglobulin (SIg) positive; Burkitt lymphoma, plasmacytoma, abdominal mass lesion	B-like
Sheep erythrocyte (sE) rosette positive; anterior mediastinal (thymic) mass lesion	T-like
Absence of cell surface markers; bone marrow involvement with no masses	"Null"

in children with and without GDID. In the group of "unselected" children, the percent distribution showed a B-like phenotype for 9 of the 79 tumors (12%), a T-like phenotype for 14 (18%), and in 56 (70%) tumors no markers were present for either B-like or T-like phenotype. Children with GDID, in whom there was adequate information available on 37 tumors, had a very different pattern; B-like phenotypes predominate with 28 of the 37 tumors (78%); the remaining 8 tumors could be defined as T-like in phenotype. No cases have been reported to the registry of a "null" cell malignancy based on surface-marker studies of the malignant blasts.

In conclusion, the significance of the comparison of non-Hodgkin lymphoproliferative malignancies in children with and without documented genetically determined immunodeficiency diseases, may be summarized in the following 2 points: 1) Children with GDID develop lymphoproliferative malignancies of T or B phenotype which present as *lymphomas;* in contrast, children without GDID (unselected children) have malignancies of a "null" phenotype which present as *leukemias.* 2) B-phenotype malignancies are more frequent in children with GDID than they are in unselected children.

TABLE 4. Percent Distribution of Leukemias and Non-Hodgkin Lymphomas by Lymphocyte Phenotype in Children 0–19 Years of Age

Phenotype	Unselected children[a]		Children with GDID[b]	
	(%)	No.	(%)	No.
B-like	12	(9)	78	(29)
T-like	18	(14)	22	(8)
"Null"	70	(56)	0	(0)

[a]Surface markers define human lymphoid malignancies with differing prognoses [3, p 18].
[b]From Immunodeficiency-Cancer Registry.

REFERENCES

1. Kersey JH, Spector BD, Good RA: Primary immunodeficiency diseases and cancer: The Immunodeficiency-Cancer Registry. Int J Cancer 12:333–347, 1973.
2. Young JL, Miller RW: Incidence of malignant tumors in US children. J Pediatr 86: 254–258, 1975.

3. Kersey J, Coccia P, Bloomfield C, Nesbit M, McKenna R, Brunning R, Hallgren H, Gajl-Peczalska K: Surface markers define human lymphoid malignancies with differing prognoses. In Thierfelder S, Rodt H, Thiel E (eds): "Immunological Diagnosis of Leukemias and Lymphomas, Haematology and Blood Transfusions." Berlin: Springer-Verlag, 1977, vol 20, pp 12–24.
4. Fudenberg HH, Good RA, Goodman HC, Hitzig W, Kunkel HG, Roitt IM, Rosen FS, Rowe DS, Seligmann M, Soothill J: Primary immunodeficiencies. Bull WHO 45:125–142, 1971.
5. Cooper M, Faulk W, Fudenberg HH, Good RA, Hitzig WA, Kunkel HG, Rosen FS, Seligmann M, Soothill J, Wedgwood RJ: Classification of primary immunodeficiencies. N Engl J Med 288:966–967, 1973.
6. Kirkpatrick CH: Cancer in immunodeficiency diseases. In Bergsma D, Schimke RN (eds): "Cancer and Genetics." New York: Alan R Liss for The National Foundation–March of Dimes, BD:OAS XII(1):61–78, 1976.

Cross Reactivity Between Hepatitis B Surface Antigen and a Male–Associated Antigen*

Jean S. Drew, AB, W. Thomas London, MD, Edward D. Lustbader, PhD, and Baruch S. Blumberg, MD, PhD

Hepatitis B surface antigen (HBsAg) is the outer coat of the Dane particle, the presumed virion of the hepatitis B virus (HBV). Both Dane particles and excess surface coat (HBsAg) particles (Fig. 1) are found in the blood of patients with acute and chronic hepatitis B. When infected with hepatitis B virus, an individual may respond by developing acute hepatitis; HBsAg appears in his blood, his serum transaminase level rises dramatically, and he may become jaundiced. This is followed by the development of antibody against HBsAg (anti-HBs) and the resolution of the viremia and clinical symptoms. In some cases, however, people become chronically infected with HBV, with little evidence of liver damage and few clinical symptoms. Many of these people do not develop anti-HBs, and they may be HBsAg(+) for years [1]. Such people are termed "chronic carriers" of HBV. They may infect other uninfected persons and apparently are at increased risk of developing certain chronic liver diseases such as chronic aggressive and chronic persistent hepatitis, postnecrotic cirrhosis, and primary hepatocellular carcinoma [2].

High frequencies of HBsAg carriers have been observed in various primarily tropical areas (West Africa, Asia, Southern Europe, Oceania [3]) and in certain disease populations (patients with leukemia, lepromatous leprosy, Down syndrome, end-stage renal disease [4–6]. In most populations studied, HBsAg is detected more often in men than in women [7–20]. Similarly, both postnecrotic cirrhosis

*This work was supported by USPHS grants CA-06551, RR-05539 and CA-06927 from the National Institutes of Health and by an appropriation from the Commonwealth of Pennsylvania.

Birth Defects: Original Article Series, Volume XIV, Number 6A, pages 91–101

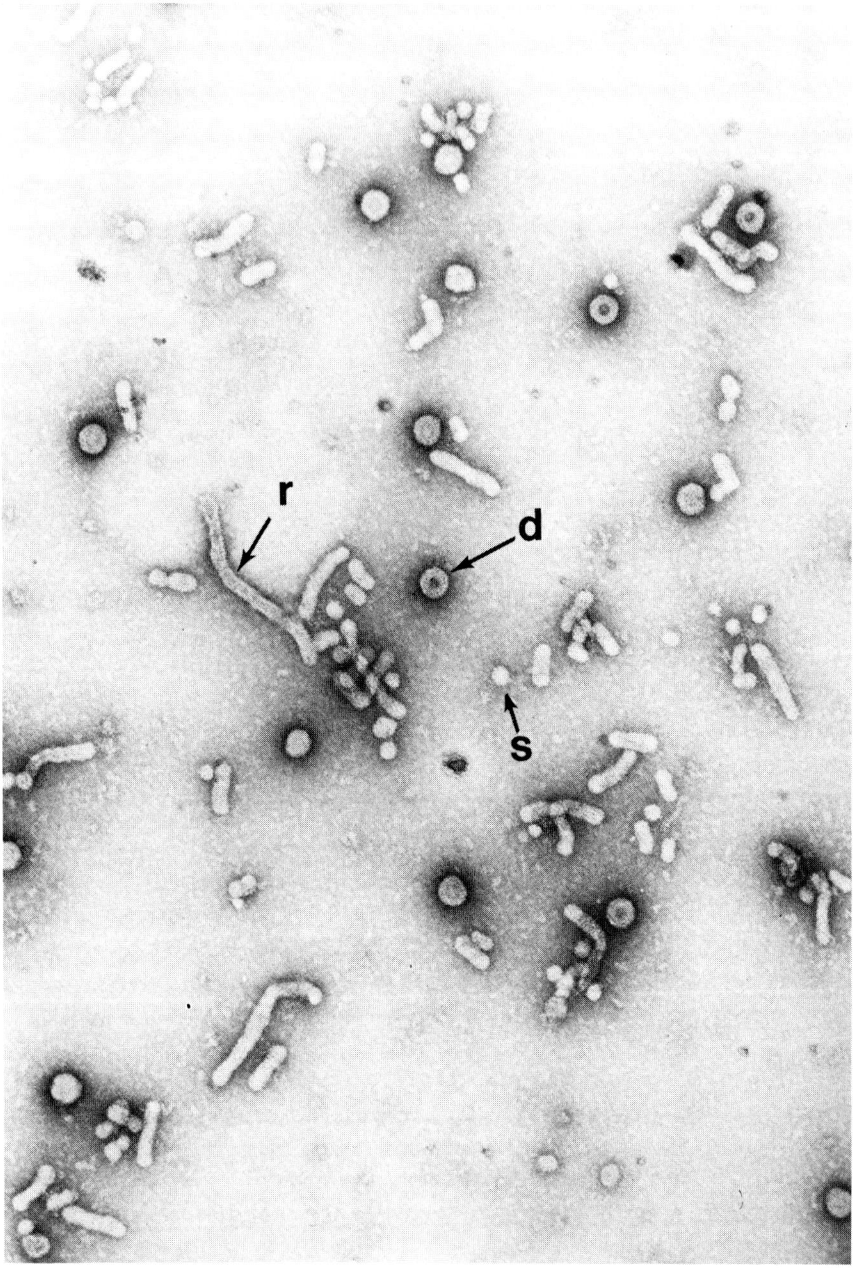

Fig. 1. HBsAg isolated from the serum of a patient with chronic hepatitis B. Particles exhibiting three morphologic forms are observed: spherical particles (s) 22 nm in diameter, rod-shaped forms (r) 22 nm in width but of varying length, and double-shelled (Dane) particles 45 nm in diameter (d). All 3 of these particles have HBsAg determinants on their surfaces. Magnification × 125,000. Electron micrograph by Halpern and Weng.

and primary hepatocellular carcinoma are more common in men [21–25], and although some forms of chronic hepatitis are more common in women HBsAg(+) chronic hepatitis is more common in men [26–27].

Some investigators have suggested that the preponderance of men among carriers and patients with chronic liver disease is due mainly to a sex difference in exposure to HBV [28]. This may not be the only explanation. We propose an additional mechanism. Last year we observed that kidney graft recipients with anti-HBs had early rejection of grafts whereas those with HBsAg had prolonged survival [29]. Knowledge of the role of male-associated antigens in the rejection of skin grafts in mice led us to the hypothesis that male cells share or cross-react with an antigen on the surface of HBV. Such cross-reactivity would render men more tolerant to the virus. We now have three kinds of evidence in support of this hypothesis. 1) Among patients with end-stage renal disease treated with chronic hemodialysis, men are more likely to become chronic carriers of HBV than women. 2) Kidney grafts from male donors survive for a much shorter time in recipients with anti-HBs than in chronic carriers of HBsAg or "uninfected" recipients. 3) The proportion of male offspring is significantly greater in families in which one or both parents are HBsAg(+) than in families in which neither parent is HBsAg(+) and one or both are anti–HBs(+). As we shall show, all three observations can be explained by the cross-reactivity hypothesis.

Greater Male Susceptibility to Chronic HBV Infection Among Renal Dialysis Patients

In most studies it is difficult to determine whether sex differences in prevalences of HBsAg and anti-HBs are due to differences in exposure or response to HBV. We have controlled the exposure variable by studying the persistence of HBsAg and development of anti-HBs among renal dialysis patients, all of whom became infected with HBV while receiving treatment at a single hemodialysis clinic [30]. Of 160 patients who began treatment without evidence of previous HBV infection, 77 subsequently became HBsAg(+). We used an adaptation of a life table analysis to compare the persistence of HBsAg by sex. Figure 2 shows the probability of remaining HBsAg(+) persistently once a patient has been HBsAg(+) for N months. Men were significantly more likely to become chronic carriers than women. Conversely, women were significantly more likely to develop anti-HBs than men. These differences were not due to sex differences in age, underlying renal disease, or rate of infection.

Early Rejection of Kidney Grafts From Male Donors by Anti-HBs(+) Patients

Many chronic renal failure patients receive renal transplants. We studied the survival of 87 grafts in 79 patients whose responses to HBV infection prior to transplantation were known [29]. Patients with anti-HBs had significantly poorer graft survival ($p < 0.05$) than either chronic carriers or "uninfected" [HBsAg(–)/

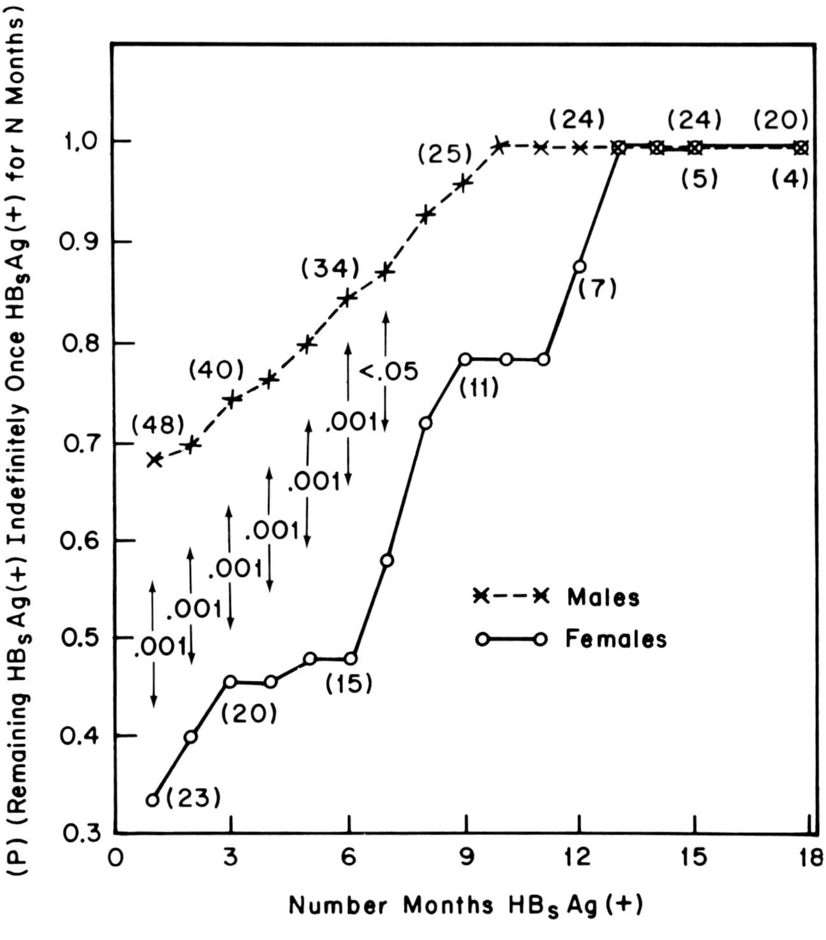

Fig. 2. The probability of male or female patients remaining HBsAg(+) persistently once detected positive for N months. The numbers in parentheses are the numbers of patients at risk at each time interval. A male dialysis patient who is HBsAg(+) on a single test has a 68% chance of remaining HBsAg(+) persistently whereas the probability for a female patient is 33%. The longer a patient is HBsAg(+) the greater his or her chance of remaining HBsAg(+). . The P values for differences between the curves were calculated by the method of Thomas and Grunkemeier [41].

anti-HBs(–)] patients. This difference was not related to factors previously known to affect graft survival, ie preformed anti-HLA antibody, HLA matching, or donor source (related vs cadaver). We found that the difference was due mainly to poor survival of grafts from male donors. Figure 3 shows graft survival among recipients without preformed anti-HLA antibody who received HLA nonidentical grafts from male donors. By 4 months after transplantation the probability of graft survival

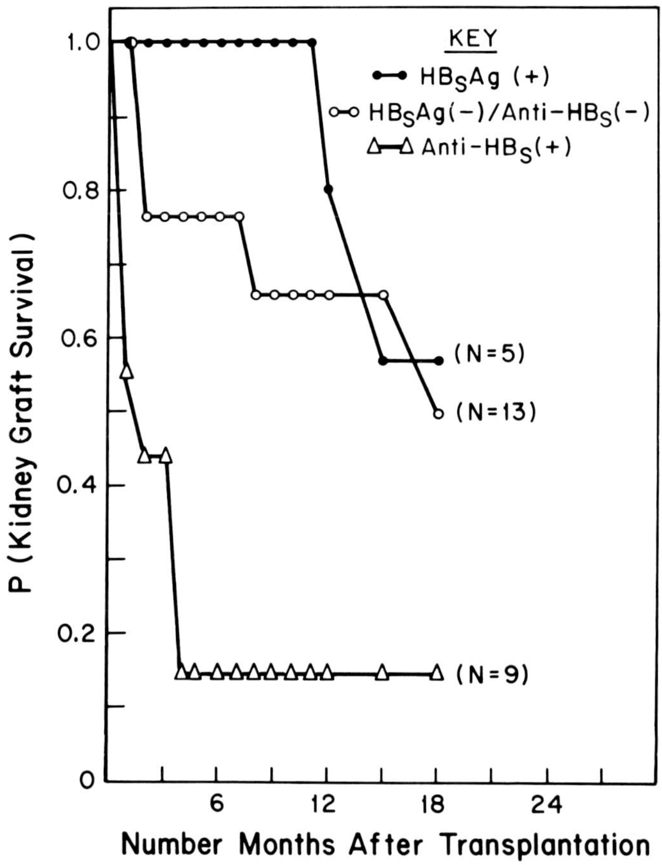

Fig.3. Kidney graft survival curves for patients who were HBsAg(+), "uninfected" [HBsAg(−)/anti-HBs(−)], or anti-HBs(+) before transplantation. Recipients did not have preformed anti-HLA antibodies and received HLA-nonidentical kidneys. The following P values for the differences between the curves were calculated by the method of Thomas and Grunkemeier [41]: HBsAg(+) vs uninfected: $p < 0.05$ at 2 and 7 months, < 0.02 at 11 months; uninfected vs anti-HBs(+): $p < 0.01$ at 1 month and at 4–15 months; HBsAg(+) vs anti-HBs(+): $p < 0.01$ at 1–12 months.

was less than 15% in anti-HBs(+) recipients, whereas at 11 months it was still 65% in uninfected recipients and 100% in HBsAg(+) recipients. Among the few patients who received grafts from female donors, there were no significant differences in graft survival between HBsAg(+), "uninfected" and anti-HBs(+) patients. Sex of the recipient was not related to these observations. The data suggest that the presence of anti-HBs prior to transplantation may be related to, or influence, a patient's response to male tissue antigens on allografts.

Association of Parents' Response to HBV With Proportion of Male Offspring

HBV may be transmitted from parents to offspring in utero or soon after birth. Infection with HBV early in life may increase the likelihood of becoming a chronic carrier of the virus [31], and vertical transmission from mother to child has been implicated as a major mechanism for the establishment of carriers in some populations [32]. Transmission from father to child, however, has not been well documented [33, 34].

Previous studies by Robertson [35] and Mazzur [36] have suggested an association between hepatitis infection and high sex ratios (the number of males ÷ the number of females × 100). In 1975, Hesser et al studied a population from Plati, a Greek village in Southern Macedonia, and found a high sex ratio of live births associated with HBsAg in parents [37, 38]. We have further analyzed the data from this study, taking into account the presence of anti-HBs as well as HBsAg in parents [39]. Sera and reproductive histories were obtained from 326 wives and 248 husbands. The sex ratio of live births was significantly higher when mothers were HBsAg(+) as opposed to anti-HBs(+) ($p = 0.022$), and when fathers were HBsAg(+) as opposed to HBsAg(–)/anti-HBs(–) ($p = 0.029$) or anti-HBs(+) ($p = 0.036$). After excluding parents with HBsAg/anti-HBs complexes or with incomplete test results, we were able to categorize 216 couples according to host response to HBV in both parents. Table 1 shows that the sex ratio of live births was highest in families in which either parent was HBsAg(+)/anti-HBs(–) [HBsAg(+) couples], intermediate in families in which both parents were HBsAg(–)/anti-HBs(–), and lowest in families in which both parents were HBsAg(–) and either or both parents were anti-HBs(+) [anti-HBs(+) couples]. A sex ratio of 145.7 seems extreme for the HBsAg(–)/anti-HBs(–) "control" group, but the 95% confidence limits of 95.7–230.0 for this ratio includes the "normal" range for

TABLE 1. Number of Male and Female Live Births According to Parents' Response to HBV

Parents' response to HBV	Number of couples	Live Births		Sex[a] ratio
		Male	Female	
Either parent HBsAg(+)/anti-HBs(–)	33	60 1.82 ± 0.22[b]	24 0.73 ± 0.11	250.0
Both parents HBsAg(–)/anti-HBs(–)	29	51 1.76 ± 0.24	35 1.21 ± 0.23	145.7
Both parents HBsAg(–) Either parent anti-HBs(+)	154	241 1.56 ± 0.10	222[c] 1.44 ± 0.10[d]	108.6

[a] [(Number of males)/(Number of females)] × 100

[b] Number of live births per couple, mean ± S.E.

[c] $2 \times 2\ \chi^2$ for HBsAg(+) vs anti-HBs(+) couples; $\chi^2 = 10.02$; $p = 0.002$ [43].

[d] Mann-Whitney U test for number of daughters born to HBsAg(+) vs anti-HBs(+) couples $p = 0.0007$

secondary sex ratios (104–107). The corresponding limits for the sex ratio of children of HBsAg(+) couples (161.1–429.1) do not include the normal range. These sex ratios reflected differences in the number of daughters, but not in the number of sons per family.

Data on birth and pregnancy order and maternal and paternal ages were available for ~ 90% of the 633 children reported. Figure 4 shows that, even while controlling such factors, HBsAg(+) couples had consistently higher proportions of male live births than anti-HBs(+) couples. These overall differences were significant. Thus it appears that HBsAg in parents is associated with a high proportion while anti-HBs in parents is associated with a low proportion of male offspring.

These three observations could all be explained by the hypothesis that there is an antigen on male cells which cross-reacts with HBsAg. This cross-reactivity would make males more likely to recognize HBsAg as "self" and therefore tolerate the antigen (ie become chronic carriers). Conversely, females would be more likely to recognize HBsAg as "nonself," and produce anti-HBs.

In kidney graft recipients, tolerance to HBsAg would result in tolerance of male tissues and thus long-term survival of grafts from male donors. Anti-HBs in a recipient, however, would react with male antigens on allografts resulting in early rejection of grafts from male donors. We can speculate that tolerance to HBsAg in potential mothers would result in lack of sensitization against male tissues and better survival of male fetuses. Anti-HBs would react with male antigens and thus hinder fertilization by Y-bearing sperm, interfere with implantation of male embryos or increase the probability of spontaneous abortion of male fetuses. Finally, HBsAg(+) carrier fathers would have HBsAg in their semen, which conceivably could protect Y-bearing sperm from anti-HBs or other cross-reacting ("antimale") antibodies in their spouses' reproductive tracts.

The biologic interactions of HBV antigens with male antigens cannot explain all the observations from the Greek study, however. If the male-associated effects of HBsAg and anti-HBs were the only factors modifying sex ratio, HBsAg(+) couples would have more sons than anti-HBs(+) couples. The observations that HBsAg(+) couples had the same number of sons but fewer daughters per family than anti-HBs(+) couples (Table 1) suggests that human behavior may interact with the effects of hepatitis B infection. In this community most younger women preferred small families and practiced some form of birth control. Also, in some parts of Greece a preference for sons (as observed in many other societies) has been reported [40]. It is possible that parents chose to limit family size only after bearing a desired number of sons. If this were so, anti-HBs(+) couples might give birth to several daughters before achieving the desired number of sons while HBsAg(+) couples would have the desired number of sons early in marriage and, as a result, restrict the number of subsequent births and therefore the total number of daughters born.

In addition to the sex polymorphism, other genetic polymorphisms may be involved in the variety of host responses to HBV infection. First, the virus itself has polymorphic antigenic determinants which behave as alleles. There is a common determinant "a" and two pairs of determinants, d or y, and w or r, which are allelic (ie one or the other, but rarely both or neither are present on each viral

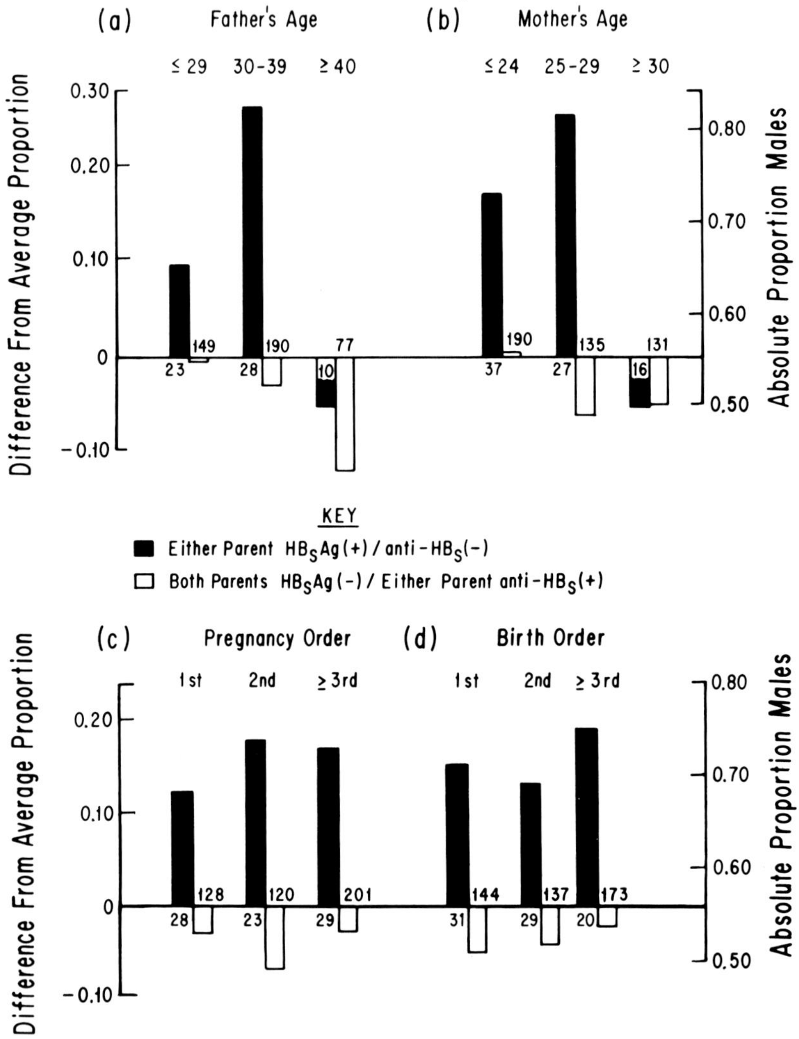

Fig. 4. Proportion of male live births according to parents' response to HBV, a) paternal and b) maternal ages, and c) pregnancy and d) birth orders. Total numbers of children are indicated. Baseline is the proportion of males among all 633 children. Z and P values (2-tailed) calculated according to the method of Mantel and Haenszel [42] are as follows: a) Z = 2.759; p = 0.006, b) Z = 3.088; p = 0.002, c) Z = 3.187; p = 0.001, d) Z = 3.207; p = 0.001.

particle). These determinants have well-defined geographic distributions. The usual antigens in Japan, China, and Korea are d and r, whereas y and w are the most common antigens in Africa, the Middle East, and the Mediterranean area, and d and w are the most frequent determinants in northern and western Europe. The most common HBs antigenic complex is ayw in the renal dialysis patients, the renal transplant patients, and the Greek populations reported here. Therefore, in each of these studies, one or a combination of these determinants may be involved in the cross-reactivity suggested. We can speculate that there is an interaction of the polymorphism of the virus and the polymorphic determinant in the host. In fact, preliminary studies of populations in which adr is the predominant HBsAg subtype complex suggest that this specificity is associated with a sex ratio distortion in the opposite direction from the one we observed in Greece.

Secondly, the male-associated cross-reacting antigen may also be polymorphic. Not all males become chronic carriers; some develop anti-HBs. Various combinations of HBsAg and host antigenic determinants could account for the variety of responses to HBV, including the preponderance of males among patients with HBV-related chronic liver diseases.

REFERENCES

1. London WT, Drew JS, Lustbader ED, Werner BG, Blumberg BS: Host responses to hepatitis B infection in patients in a chronic hemodialysis unit. Kidney Int 12:51,1977.
2. Blumberg BS, Larouzé B, London WT, Werner B, Hesser JE, Millman I, Saimot G, Payet M: The relation of infection with the hepatitis B agent to primary hepatic carcinoma. Am J Pathol 81:669–682, 1975.
3. Blumberg BS, Gerstley BJS, Hungerford DA, London WT, Sutnick AI: A serum antigen (Australia antigen) in Down syndrome, leukemia, and hepatitis. Ann Intern Med 66:924–931, 1967.
4. Blumberg BS, Melartin L, Lechat M, Guinto RS: Association between lepromatous leprosy and Australia antigen. Lancet 2:173–176, 1967.
5. Sutnick AI, London WT, Gerstley BJS, Cronlund MM, Blumberg BS: Anicteric hepatitis associated with Australia antigen. Occurrence in patients with Down's syndrome. JAMA 205:670–674, 1968.
6. London WT, DiFiglia M, Sutnick AI, Blumberg BS: An epidemic of hepatitis in a chronic hemodialysis unit. Australia antigen and difference in host response. N Engl J Med 281:571–578, 1969.
7. Blumberg BS, Melartin L, Guinto RA, Werner B: Family studies of a human serum isoantigen system (Australia antigen). Am J Hum Genet 18:594–608, 1966.
8. Szmuness W, Hirsch RL, Prince AM, Levine RM, Harley EJ, Ikram H: Hepatitis B surface antigen in blood donors. Further observations. J Infect Dis 131:111–118, 1975.
9. Szmuness W, Prince A, Brotman B, Hirsch R: Hepatitis B antigen and antibody in blood donors: An epidemiologic study. J Infect Dis 127:17–25, 1973.
10. Klinman A, Reid NR, Lilly C, Morrison J: Hepatitis associated antigen (Australia antigen) in Massachusetts blood donors. N Engl J Med 285:783–785, 1971.
11. Farrow LJ, Lamb SG, Coghill NF, Lindon RL, Preece J, Zuckerman AJ, Stewart JS: Hepatitis B antigen in viral hepatitis in West London. Br Med J 3:83–86, 1974.

12. Soulier JP, Courouce-Pauty AM, Benamon-Djiane D: Study of the Australia antigen and of the corresponding antibody in blood donors in Paris. Vox Sang 19:345–351, 1970.
13. Terrier E, Simonneau M, Jaulmes B: Screening blood donors for Australia antigen carriers at the Broussais Hospital. Vox Sang 19:352–356, 1970.
14. Okochi K, Mayumi M, Haguino Y, Saito N: Evaluation of frequency of Australia antigen in blood donors of Tokyo by means of immune adherence hemagglutination technique. Vox Sang 19:332–337, 1970.
15. Blumberg BS, Sutnick AI, London WT, Melartin L: Sex distribution of Australia antigen. Arch Intern Med 130:227–231, 1972.
16. Lous P, Skinhoj P, Olsen H: HAA-antigen determination in 12,000 patients in a general Copenhagen hospital. Vox Sang 19:379–383, 1970.
17. Blumberg BS, Melartin L, LeChat M, Guinto RA: Association between lepromatous leprosy and Australia antigen. Lancet 2:173–176, 1967.
18. Leski M, Grivaux C, Courouce-Pauty AM: Australia antigen in hemodialysis and renal transplantation units. Vox Sang 19:359–368, 1970.
19. Goodman M, Wainwright RL, Weir HF, Gall JC: A sex difference in the carrier state of Australia (hepatitis associated) antigen. Pediatrics 48:907–913, 1971.
20. Szmuness W, Prince AM, Etling GF, Pick R: Development and distribution of hemagglutinating antibody against the hepatitis B antigen in institutionalized populations. J Infect Dis 126:498–506, 1972.
21. Larouzé B, London WT, Saimot G, Werner BG, Lustbader ED, Payet M, Blumberg BS: Host responses to hepatitis B infection in patients with primary hepatic carcinoma and their families. Lancet 2:534–538, 1976.
22. Tong MJ, Sun S-C, Schaeffer BT, Chang N-K, Lo K-J, Peters RL: Hepatitis associated antigen and hepatocellular carcinoma in Taiwan. Ann Intern Med 75:687–691, 1971.
23. Larouzé B, London WT, Saimot G, Werner BG, Lustbader ED, Payet M, Blumberg BS: Host responses to hepatitis B infection in patients with primary hepatic carcinoma and their families. A case/control study in Senegal, West Africa. Lancet 2:534–538, 1976.
24. Vogel CL, Anthony PP, Sadikali F, Barker LF, Peterson MR: Hepatitis associated antigen and antibody in hepatocellular carcinoma: Results of a continuing study. J Natl Cancer Inst 48:1583–1588, 1972.
25. Vogel CL, Anthony PP, Mody N, Barker LF: Hepatitis associated antigen in Ugandan patients with hepatocellular carcinoma. Lancet 2:621–624, 1970.
26. Shulman NR: Hepatitis associated antigen. Am J Med 49:669–692, 1970.
27. Bulkley BH, Heizer WD, Goldfinger SE, Isselbacher KJ, Shulman NR: Distinctions in chronic active hepatitis based on circulating hepatitis-associated antigen. Lancet 2:1323–1326, 1970.
28. Mazzur S, Jones N: Equal susceptibility of male and females on Santa Cruz Island to the carrier state of hepatitis B surface antigen. J Infect Dis 133:331–333, 1976.
29. London WT, Drew JS, Blumberg BS, Grossman RA, Lyons PJ: Infection in patients with kidney transplants. N Engl J Med 296:241–244, 1977.
30. London WT, Drew JS: Sex differences in response to hepatitis B infection among patients receiving chronic dialysis treatment. Proc Natl Acad Sci USA 74:2561, 1977.
31. Bruyns C, Urbain-Vansanten G, Planard C, DeVos-Cloeteus C, Urbain J: Ontogeny of mouse B lymphocytes and inactivation by antigen of early B lymphocytes. Proc Natl Acad Sci USA 73:2462–2466, 1976.
32. Nishioka K: Discussion. Viral hepatitis: Epidemiology. In "Proceedings of a Symposium on Viral Hepatitis." National Academy of Sciences, Washington, DC. Thorofare, NJ: Charles B. Slack, 1975, p 322.

33. Mazzur S, Blumberg BS, Friedlaender JS: Silent maternal transmission of Australia antigen. Nature 247:41–43, 1974.
34. Blumberg BS: Australia antigen. A review with comments on maternal effect. Bull Acad Med Toronto 45:45–51, 1972.
35. Robertson JS, Sheard AV: Altered sex ratio after an outbreak of hepatitis. Lancet 1:532–534, 1973.
36. Mazzur S, Watson TM: Excess males among siblings of Australia antigen carriers. Nature 250:60–61, 1974.
37. Hesser JE, Economidou J, Blumberg BS: Hepatitis B surface antigen, fertility and sex ratio: Implications for health planning. Hum Biol 47:415–425, 1975.
38. Hesser JE, Blumberg BS, Drew JS: Hepatitis B surface antigen, fertility and sex ratio: Implications for health planning. Hum Biol 48:73–81, 1976.
39. Drew JS, London WT, Lustbader ED, Blumberg BS: Association of response to hepatitis B virus in parents with sex of offspring. (In preparation)
40. Hesser JE: Infectious disease and population dynamics. Australia antigen (HBsAg) in parents, sex ratio of offspring and fertility. Studies in an Agrarian Village of Greek Macedonia, Doctoral Thesis, Department of Anthropology, University of Pennsylvania, 1974.
41. Thomas DR, Grunkemeier GL: Confidence interval estimation of survival probabilities for censored data. J Am Stat Assoc 70:865–871, 1975.
42. Mantel N, Haenszel W: Statistical aspects of the analysis of data from retrospective studies of disease. J Natl Cancer Inst 22:719–748, 1959.
43. Siegel S: "Nonparametric Statistics for the Behavioral Sciences." New York: McGraw-Hill 1956, pp 116–127.

Short Stature, Absent Thumbs, Flat Facies, Anosmia and Combined Immune Deficiency (CID)

M. H. K. Shokeir, MD, PhD

NTRODUCTION

Absence of thumbs has been noted in several disorders with varying frequency. In poikiloderma congenita (Rothmund-Thomson syndrome), absence or hypoplasia of thumbs may be noted along with the better known features of cutaneous involvement, zonular cataract and corneal dystrophy [1–3]. In the radial aplasia-thrombocytopenia syndrome, the radius is hypoplastic or even absent. The thumb is also affected, albeit to a lesser extent. The thrombocytopenia is associated with other hematologic manifestations such as granulocytosis, eosinophilia, and anemia that cannot be entirely ascribed to excessive bleeding. It is the megakaryocytes, however, which bear the brunt of the disease, and are either absent or functionally inactive [4–6]. In the Fanconi pancytopenia syndrome, in addition to the pancytopenia, short stature, hypogonadism, and splenic hypoplasia, the thumbs may be hypoplastic [7, 8]. The chromosomes are known to manifest excessive breakage in this disorder as well [9]. In the Roberts syndrome [10–12] absence of the thumbs may occur as a feature of the generalized and major skeletal dysplasia and hypomelia which may reach phocomelic proportions. These four disorders are inherited in an autosomal recessive fashion, with a notable ethnic variation.

In the Holt-Oram syndrome, absence of thumbs is a rare occurrence, hypoplasia and nonopposability being the rule. Cardiac lesions, particularly ventricular and atrial septal defects [13], and hypoplastic clavicles are the other characteristic features of the disorder, which is inherited in an autosomal dominant fashion [14].

To our knowledge absence of thumbs in association with other skeletal manifestations, combined immune deficiency (CID), ichthyosiform dermatosis, and variable congenital cardiac lesions has hitherto not been described. In this com-

Birth Defects: Original Article Series, Volume XIV, Number 6A, pages 103–116

munication we wish to report this association in 9 individuals (4 males and 5 females) distributed in 5 sibships from 3 separate families of 2 distinct ethnic origins. The distribution of affected individuals in their respective kindreds and the consanguinity among the parents of some of them are compatible with autosomal recessive inheritance.

PRESENT INVESTIGATIONS

Nine cases have been ascertained with the condition outlined in the present work. The proposita of *Case 1,* in whom the expression appears to represent a prototype of the disorder, will be described in detail. The manifestations observed in the other propositi and the related affected individuals will be briefly noted.

Case 1 (Fig. 1) is a 38-year-old single white woman who presented because of skin lesions dating as far back as age 3 and recurrent respiratory tract, urinary

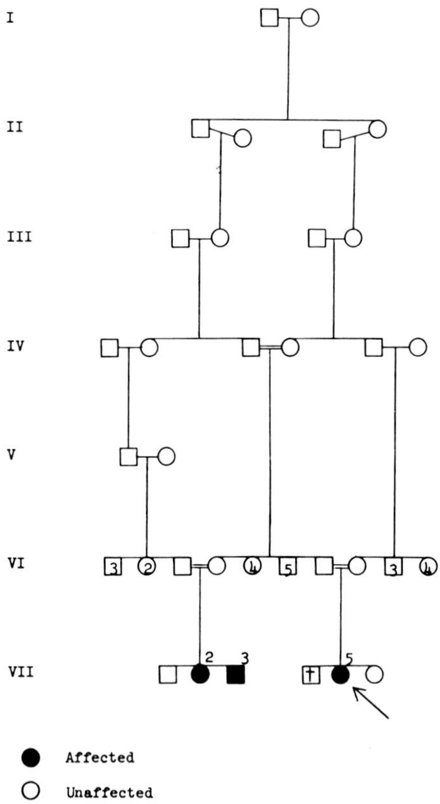

Fig. 1. Pedigree of family in *Case 1.* Note consanguinity.

tract, middle ear, and eye infections. She also had several episodes of pleurisy and had suffered a protracted attack of pertussis at 2 years of age that lasted for 14 months. Her history of recurrent respiratory tract infections was heralded at 6 months of age by a severe episode of pneumonia that was very slow to resolve and was followed by pleurisy.

On physical examination, the patient was cooperative and of normal intellect. She was well proportioned but very short in stature, measuring 133 cm in height, and weighing 29 kg. Her hair was coarse, sparse, and brittle. Her head was small but proportionate to her size. Her facial features were flat (Fig. 2) with a depressed nasal bridge and short palpebral fissures. She had virtually no eyelashes or eyebrows. Her lid margins showed evidence of chronic blepharitis and meibomianitis. Her ocular examination revealed small cornea and chronic conjunctivitis but was otherwise unremarkable; in particular she had no corneal dystrophy or zonular lenticular cataract. There was, however, evidence of chronic suppura-

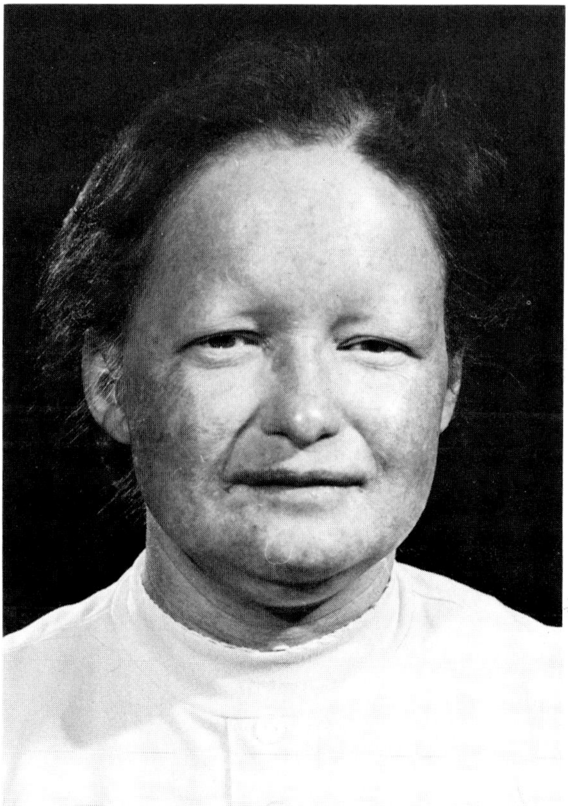

Fig. 2. Photograph of proposita of *Case 1*, showing characteristic facies.

tive infection of the lacrimal system. Her palate was somewhat high-arched but her teeth were unremarkable. The mucous lining of both the mouth and the tongue showed evidence of candida infection. There were mouth ulcerations which the patient described as a practically perpetual ailment. Although both her vision and hearing were largely preserved, she had no sense of smell (anosmia). Her auricles were unremarkable, but middle ear examination disclosed evidence of chronic otitis media. She had a moderate degree of hearing loss in the right ear, presumably due to chronic otitis media.

Chest, cardiac, and abdominal examinations were unremarkable. The patient had normal breast development and adequate axillary and pubic hair growth (menarche had occurred at 14 years of age).

The skin displayed widespread lesions particularly involving the limbs and not sparing the palms (Fig. 3) or soles (Fig. 4). The lesions took the form of verrucous growths with scaling, crusting, and cracking. In several spots this was complicated by what appeared to be secondary infection and mild suppuration. Both her mouth and vagina exhibited evidence of candidiasis.

On examination of the skeletal system, the most striking feature, apart from her extremely short stature, was complete absence of thumbs and the 1st metacarpal bones (Fig. 5) as well as bowing and inability to pronate or supinate

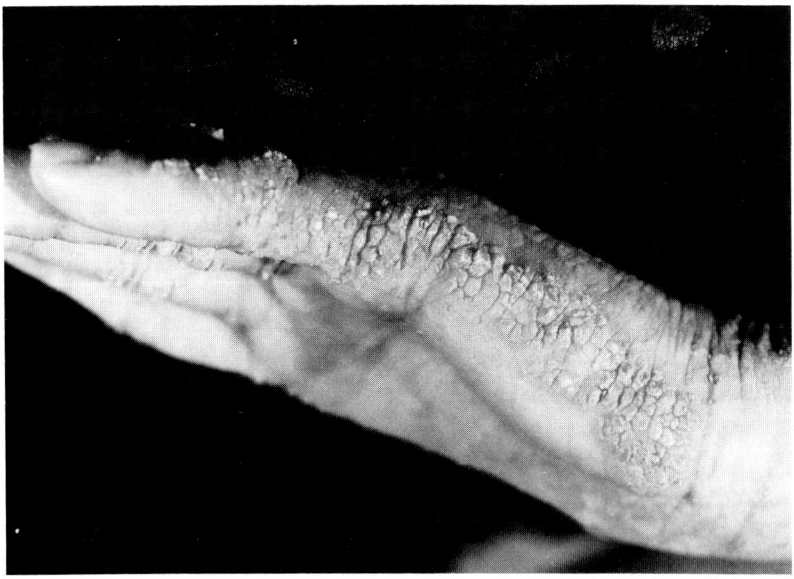

Fig. 3. Verrucous skin lesion on palm in *Case 1.*

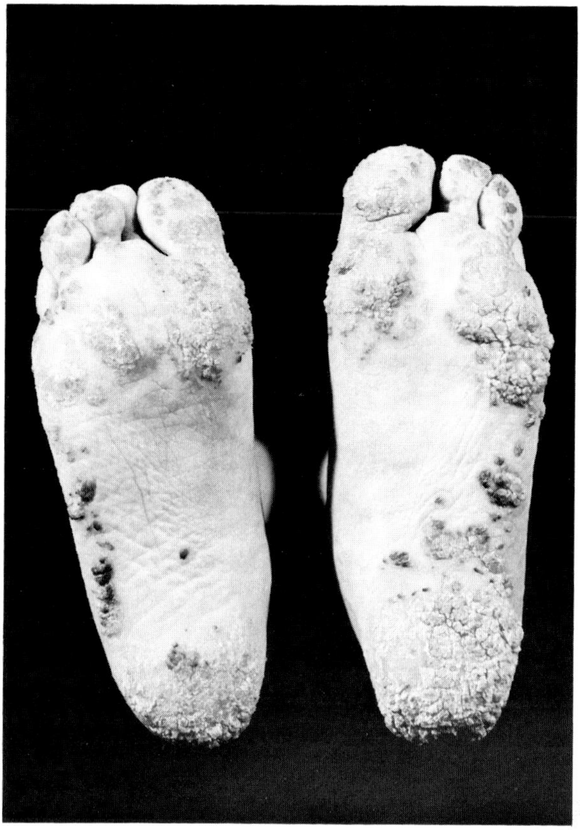

Fig. 4. Skin lesions on soles in *Case 1.*

both forearms. Her feet, however, had all the toes, and with the exception of their small size and the warty skin lesions they were unremarkable.

Investigations

Physical examination of eyes. Manifestations of blepharitis and meibomianitis were disclosed by slit-lamp examination of the lids. The lashes were practically absent. The few remaining ones were short and stubby and there was some trichiasis. Pannus formation superiorly in both corneas and slight epithelial infiltration on the right side were observed.

Radiologic examination. Osteopenia was detected in the distal portions of both humeri, radii, and ulnae as well as the foot bones bilaterally. Specific

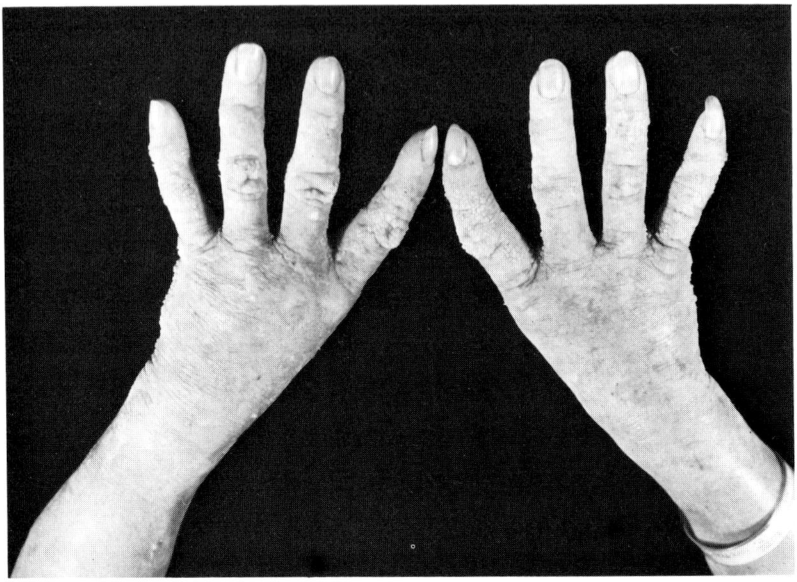

Fig. 5. Photograph of wrists and hands (*Case 1*), showing absence of thumbs.

anomalies were detected in each olecranon, which remained unfused with the body of the ulna (Fig. 6), and the right olecranon was further bisected horizontally (Fig. 7).

The ulnae were also short and bowed with posterior convexity. A linear defect (? pseudoarthrosis) was detected at the convexity (Fig. 8). The ulna projected distally beyond the distal end of radius. Whereas the proximal row of carpal bones was present, the distal one was virtually absent. In particular, the trapezium, trapezoid, and capitate bones were absent and the hamate was represented by a rudimentary bone lacking its normal hook. Both the thumb and the 1st metacarpal bones were absent bilaterally (Fig. 9). The remaining fingers were normal save for slight shortening of the index fingers.

In the lower limbs the patellae were bipartite and osteopenia in both feet was noted (Fig. 10).

Immunologic and hematologic investigations. There was evidence of generalized hypogammaglobulinemia: IgG 560 mg/dl, IgM 25 mg/dl, and complete absence of plasma IgA. IgD was not measured and IgE was less than 25 units, the normal being 350 units or less. Phytohemagglutinin (PHA) stimulation revealed a depressed T-cell response. There was mild leukopenia ($< 3{,}000$/cu mm) with un-

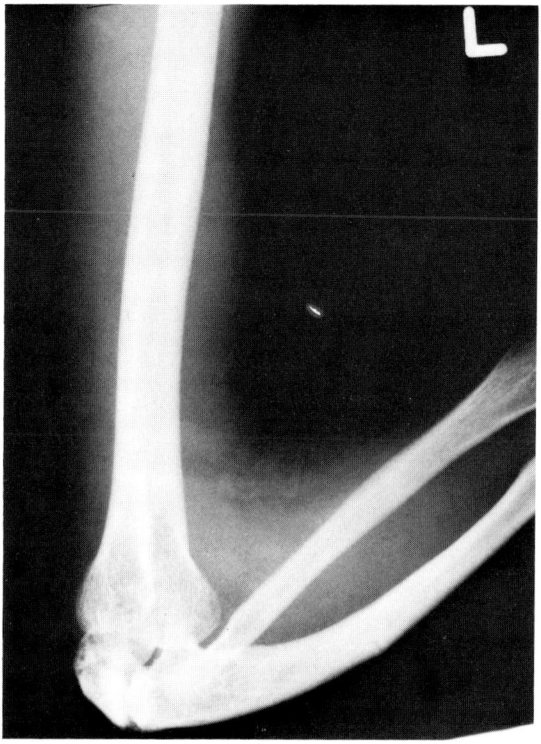

Fig. 6. X-ray film of left elbow (*Case 1*), showing unfused olecranon and pseudoarthrosis of the ulna.

remarkable differential count (polymorphonuclears 65%, eosinophils 1%, lymphocytes 27% and monocytes 7%). The platelets were adequate in number (264,000/cu mm), morphology, and function.

On lymph node biopsy there was morphologic evidence of B-cell and T-cell deficiency.

Biochemical investigations. Several enzymes which have been previously implicated in CID, such as adenosine deaminase (ADA) and nucleophosphorylase (NP) were studied in this case and no abnormalities were found.

Electrolyte and general hormone assays revealed normal values.

Cytogenetic investigations. Chromosome analysis revealed 46 chromosomes with XX sex chromosomal complement. Both G- and Q- banding patterns were normal.

The proposita, the product of a consanguineous mating, has two similarly

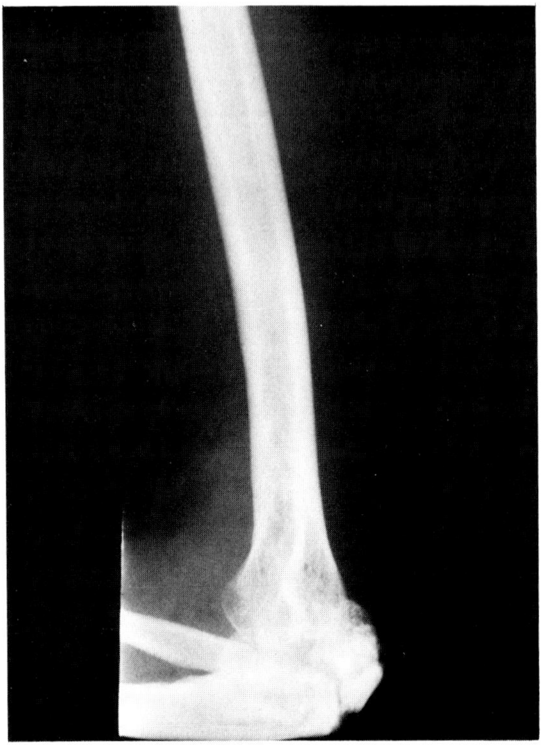

Fig. 7. X-ray film of right elbow (*Case 1*), showing unfused and bisected olecranon.

affected cousins who are themselves the product of a first-cousin marriage. They come from a small, highly inbred Rumanian-Austrian community in the Canadian prairies.

Other Cases

Case 2 (Fig. 11) is a 19-year-old white male who presented because of severe mouth ulceration. He had suffered repeated episodes of pneumonia, otitis media, gastroenteritis, pyelonephritis, and skin infections. He was born missing both thumbs and the corresponding metacarpals. At the time of presentation he measured 138 cm and weighed 35 kg. Other features included dry, woolly scalp hair, dermatosis, atrial septal defect and anosmia.

Immunologic studies revealed combined T- and B-cell function deficiency. The T-cell response to PHA stimulation was poor. The patient also had dimin-

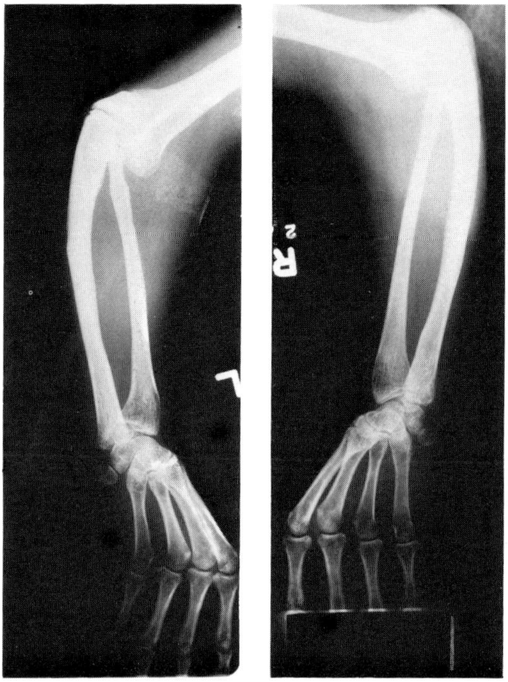

Fig. 8. X-ray film of forearms and wrists (*Case 1*), showing absence of distal row of carpals (a rudimentary hamate, however, persists).

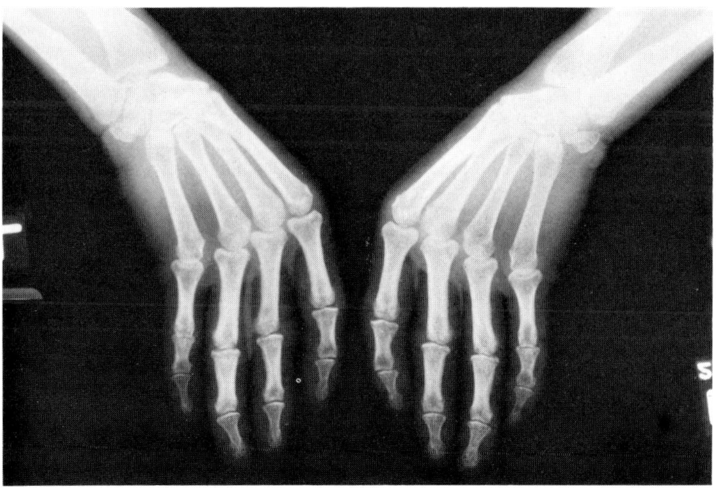

Fig. 9. X-ray film of the wrists and hands in (*Case 1*), showing deficient carpal bones and absence of 1st metacarpals and thumbs.

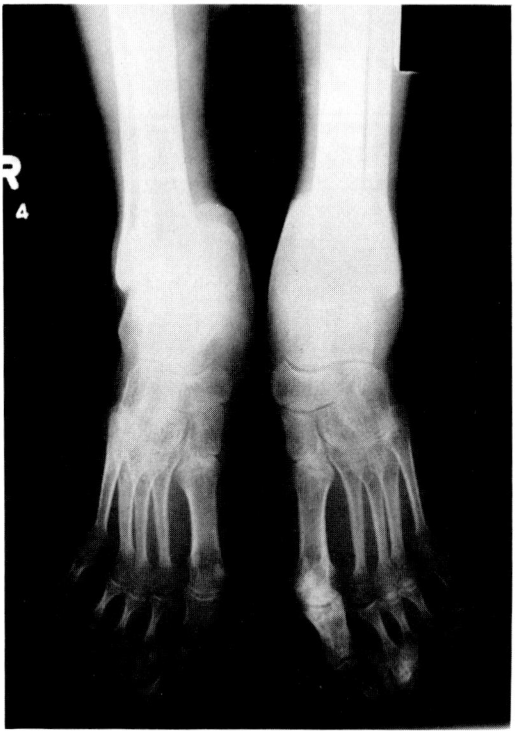

Fig. 10. X-ray film of ankles and feet (*Case 1*), showing osteopenia. Note that all 5 rays exist in both feet.

ished plasma immunoglobulin levels: IgG 400 mg/dl, IgM 10 mg/dl and absent IgA.

This patient had a similarly affected 16-year-old sister; she, however, had no detectable heart lesion. They come from a small inbred German community in the Canadian prairies.

Case 3 (Fig. 12) is a 35-year-old white male who presented because of fatigue, chest pains, palpitation, and fainting spells. He had no thumbs and had a long history of repeated respiratory, gastrointestinal, and kidney infections. He was also believed to have malabsorption syndrome. His skin had always manifested icthyosiform dermatosis. He had always been subject to repeated and painful mouth ulceration and "cheesy" secretions on the tongue. As an infant he had been the victim of such a severe attack of varicella that the diagnosis of smallpox

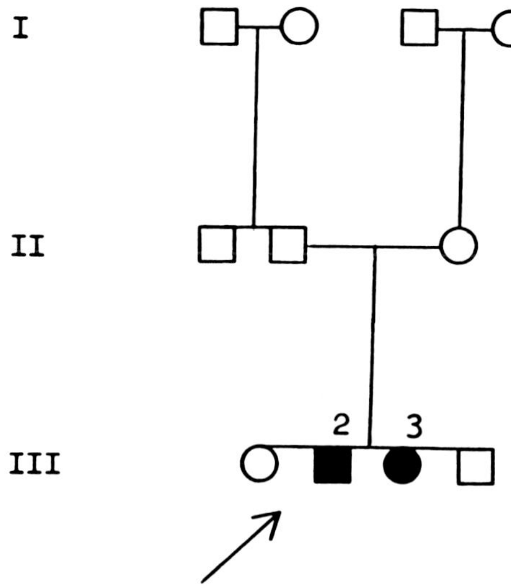

Fig. 11. Pedigree of family in *Case 2*.

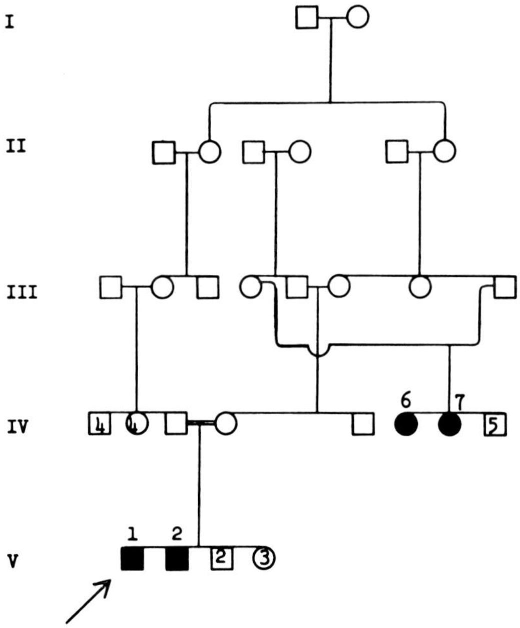

Fig. 12. Pedigree of family in *Case 3*. Note consanguinity of patient's parents.

was seriously entertained. However, he lacked the characteristic scars. He had an atrial septal defect and pulmonic stenosis.

Radiologic investigations confirmed the absence of both thumbs, 1st metacarpal bones, and distal rows of the carpal bones bilaterally.

Immunologic investigations revealed depressed T-cell function and hypogammaglobulinemia with total absence of plasma IgA.

This patient's family belongs to the same German community as the family in *Case 2.*

DISCUSSION

The cases described above share certain characteristics: normally proportioned dwarfism; absent thumbs, 1st metacarpals, and some carpal bones; anosmia and skin lesions in the form of icthyosiform dermatosis. Combined immune deficiency (CID) with increased susceptibility to bacterial, viral, and fungal infections – in particular, mucocutaneous candidiasis – was noted in differing degrees in all of them. Intellect, vision, and hearing were normally preserved. Sexual maturation was normal, although slightly delayed in onset. All of the patients, who ranged in age from 16 to 42 years, were unmarried and none had reproduced. Despite their multiple problems, none appeared in acute distress.

There was some variation regarding the incidence of congenital heart disease, which affected three of the nine patients. The lesions were atrial septal defect (ASD) and pulmonic stenosis in the patient in *Case 2,* and ASD alone in VL (*Case 3*) and in the patient in *Case 2.* Also the extent of deficiency of carpal bones varied from complete absence of the distal row of the carpals: trapezium, trapezoid, capitate and hamate, to deficiency of only the trapezium and trapezoid; or intermediate states where a rudimentary bone such as a dysplastic hamate had persisted. Although the association of absence of the thumbs and hematologic disorders, particularly thrombocytopenia or even pancytopenia, is well recognized [4–9], the presence of CID as an integral part of the manifestations is, to our knowledge, yet undescribed. Conversely, although skeletal dysplasias have been described in association with CID [15, 16], none has encompassed the spectrum of anomalies herein reported – in particular, the complete absence of the thumbs, 1st metacarpals, and the distal row of carpal bones. The brother and sister reported by Hong et al [17] are particularly intriguing since they suffered from the combinations of CID with short-limb dwarfism and skin involvement in the form of ectodermal dysplasia.

Evidence of humoral immune deficiency was elicited in all the cases herein reported. There were varying degrees of hypogammaglobulinemia but the most consistent finding was absence or near absence of plasma IgA. In all of them there was also poor T-cell response on PHA stimulation and neutropenia. Clinically all patients exhibited increased susceptibility to viral and fungal as well as pyogenic infections, which is in accord with combined T- and B-cell deficiency, respectively. The degree of CID was sufficiently severe to cause them a lifelong succession of bacterial, viral, and fungal infections. It was not so severe, however, as to preclude survival beyond infancy and childhood, as is observed in the other well-known examples of CID [17, 18].

The disorder of metaphyseal chondrodysplasia, or cartilage-hair hypoplasia [19] presents some similarity to the condition manifested by our patients. Neutropenia with abnormal cellular immunity has been reported in this disorder [20], which is also characterized by short-limb dwarfism, attributable to hypoplasia of the cartilage. The hair is sparse,fine in texture, small in caliber, and light in color. The disorder, which is also inherited in an autosomal recessive fashion, tends to cluster in certain highly inbred ethnic groups such as the Amish.

Another condition which bears some resemblance is the Rothmund-Thomson syndrome. It differs, however, in that the affected patients have hypogonadism, juvenile cataract, corneal dystrophy, and cutaneous telangiectasia with excessive pigmentation. Moreover, CID has not been reported in the above syndrome, which is inherited as an autosomal recessive.

It is not surprising that the condition described in this communication overlaps in its expression other apparently similarly inherited disorders whose phenotypic spectrum embraces skeletal, ectodermal, hematologic, and immune system involvement.

Inspection of the pedigrees of the affected individuals suggests that the operative mode of inheritance is autosomal recessive. Involvement of both sexes (4 males, 5 females), freedom of the parents from the disorder, existence of unaffected sibs, consanguinity between the parents in 3 of the 5 reported sibships, and the highly endogamous ethnic groups from which the patients came are in support of autosomal recessive inheritance. Application of the simple sib method [21] to the observed distribution of patients in their respective sibships (4 in 19) yields only insignificant departure from the 1 in 4 expectation based on the above mode of inheritance. The numbers are perhaps too small to permit meaningful conclusions from the statistical testing, but $\chi^2_{(1)} = 0.124$, $0.50 < p < 0.75$.

The multifaceted but consistent character of the disorder displayed by the patients attests to the pleiotropy of the mutant gene. This diversity of expression notwithstanding, the ultimate defect is likely but a single albeit critical defect whose precise nature is yet undefined. Doubtless, however, it involves a crucial enzymatic or other biochemical developmental step in the differentiation of the skeletal, immunologic, hematologic, and dermatologic systems.

REFERENCES

1. Rook A, Davis R, Stevanovic D: Poikiloderma congenitale. Rothmund-Thomson syndrome. Acta Derm Venerol (Stockh) 39:392, 1959.
2. Silver HK: Rothmund-Thomson syndrome: An oculocutaneous disorder. Am J Dis Child 111:182, 1966.
3. Oates RK, Lewis MB, Walker-Smith JA: The Rothmund-Thomson syndrome. Aust Paediatr J 7:103, 1971.
4. Gross H, Groh C, Weippl G: Congenitale hypoplastische thrombopenie mit radialaplaisie. Neue Osterr Z Kinderheilkd 1:574, 1956.
5. Shaw S, Oliver RAM: Congenital hypoplastic thrombocytopenia with skeletal deformities in siblings. Blood 14:374, 1956.
6. Hall JG, Levin J, Kuhn JP, Ottenheimer EJ, Van Berkum KAP, McKusick VA: Thrombocytopenia with absent radius (TAR). Medicine 48:411, 1969.
7. Fanconi G: Die familiare panmydopatline. Schweiz Med Wochenschr 94:1309, 1964.
8. Nillsson LR: Chronic pancytopenia with multiple congenital abnormalities (Fanconi's anemia) Acta Paediatr 49:518, 1960.
9. Schmid WK, Scharer K, Baumann T, Fanconi G: Chromosomen bruchigkeit bei der familiaren panmyelopathie (Typus Fanconi). Schweiz Med Wochenschr 95:1461, 1965.
10. Roberts JB: A child with double cleft of lip and palate, protrusion of the intermaxillary portion of the upper jaw and imperfect development of the bones of the four extremities. Ann Surg 70:252, 1919.
11. Herrmann J, Feingold M, Tuffli GA, Opitz JM: A familial dysmorphogenetic syndrome of limb deformities, characteristic facial appearance and associated anomalies: The "pseudothalidomide or SC-Syndrome." In Bergsma D (ed): Part III. "Limb Malformations." New York: The National Foundation–March of Dimes. BD:OAS V(3):81–89, 1969.
12. Freeman MVR, Williams DW, Schimke N, Temtamy SA: The Roberts syndrome. Clin Genet 5:1–16, 1974.
13. Holt M, Oram S: Familial heart disease with skeletal malformations. Br Heart J 22: 236–242, 1960.
14. Lewis KB, Bruce RA, Baum D, Motulsky AG: The upper limb-cardiovascular syndrome. An autosomal dominant genetic effect on embryogenesis. JAMA 193:1080–1086, 1965.
15. Alexander WJ, Dunbar JS: Unusual bone changes in thymic alymphoplasia. Ann Radiol 11:389–394, 1968.
16. Davis JA: A case of Swiss-type agammaglobulinaemia and achondroplasia. Br Med J 2:1371–1374, 1966.
17. Hong R, Gatti R, Rathburn JC, Good RA: Thymic hypoplasia and thyroid dysfunction. N Engl J Med 282:470–474, 1970.
18. Greenwood RD, Traisman HS, Rice HM, Oh-Paik SG: Swiss-type agammaglobulinemia in the United States. Autosomal recessive lymphopenic thymic dysplasia with agammaglobulinemia. Am J Dis Child 121:30–34, 1971.
19. McKusick VA, Eldridge R, Hostetler JA, Egeland JA, Ruangwit U: Dwarfism in the Amish. II. Cartilage-hair hypoplasia. Bull Johns Hopkins Hosp 116:285–326, 1965.
20. Lux SE, Johnston RB Jr, August CS, Say B, Penchaszadeh VB, Rosen FS, McKusick VA: Neutropenia and abnormal cellular immunity in cartilage-hair hypoplasia. N Engl J Med 282:234–236, 1970.
21. Weinberg W: Mathematische Grundlagen der Probandenmethode. Z Vererbungsl 48: 179–228, 1927.

antibodies and experimental thyroiditis produced in rabbits by immunization with autogenic thyroid extract [1, 2] by the presence of circulating antithyroglobulin antibodies to normal thyroid constituents in the plasma of many patients with Hashimoto thyroiditis [3] and by the demonstration of migration inhibition factor to thyroid particulate antigen and thyroid microsomal antigen in patients with thyroiditis [4, 5].

Myasthenia gravis has also been suspected to be a disorder of the immune mechanism for many years. Simpson in 1960 suggested that it might result from autoimmunization and postulated blockage by an autoantibody of the muscle receptor for acetylcholine [6]. Direct evidence of antibody to skeletal muscle was demonstrated by Strauss et al [7]. Other evidence suggesting an autoimmune pathogenesis was reviewed extensively by Abdou et al [8] and Simpson et al [9]. The most recent studies including experimental immune myasthenia gravis suggest that antibodies to acetylcholine receptor are responsible for the neuromuscular block of myasthenia gravis [10].

Association of two or more disorders presumably of autoimmune origin has been increasingly reported recently. However, reports of the association of myasthenia gravis and lymphocytic thyroiditis are relatively rare [11–19].

Repeated chromosome analysis of lymphocytes failed to demonstrate mosaicism in this patient. This phenomenon could be due to many factors, including difference in selection and pressure and sample size. Unfortunately skin or other tissue was not obtained for culture in order to show whether mosaicism was present in those tissues.

Clinical observation in this case favors the diagnosis of mosaicism because of less typical Turner phenotype with relatively well-developed breasts and regular menstruation. However, clinical delineation of the mosaic Turner syndrome can often pose problems.

The pathology of follicular lymphoid infiltration of thymic medulla seen in myasthenia gravis is similar to that of lymphocytic (Hashimoto) thyroiditis. Both Hashimoto thyroiditis and experimental autoimmune thyroiditis are shown to be accompanied by antibody to autologous thyroglobulin; furthermore, immune complexes are found between the follicular basement membrane and plasma membrane in mice [20]. Similarly, in naturally occurring myasthenia gravis and experimental autoimmune myasthenia gravis there are detectable circulating antibodies to autologous acetylcholine receptor [21, 22] and myasthenia gravis can be passively transferred to normal animals with immunoglobulin G from affected donor [23]. Lately immune complexes (IgG and C_3) have been demonstrated at the motor end-plate by an immunoperoxidase technique in myasthenia patients [24].

HLA-8 has been shown to be statistically (but not absolutely) associated with myasthenia gravis [25–32]. However, it is not a prerequisite for the occurrence of myasthenia gravis. Although HLA-8 is more commonly seen in females with early onset of the disease, Fritze et al [29] observed that HLA-3 was significantly increased in males and in patients with thymoma. Feltkamp et al [28] and Oosterhuis [33] have also observed that HLA-2 is increased in patients with thymoma or with late onset of myasthenia gravis. HLA-7, however, was found more common in males [28, 29]. Thymectomy in this patient with an HLA type of 2, 3, and 7 and without thymoma at the time of operation might be significant. Thymomas often are detected in myasthenia gravis after the fourth decade and the presence of this antigen HLA types 2, 3, and possibly 7 and the absence of HLA-8 might be helpful in distinguishing thymomatous from nonthymomatous myasthenia gravis and in identifying thymomatous from nonthymomatous myasthenics at risk for thymomas [31].

The patient has autoantibodies to at least three different types of tissues: a) thyroid, b) smooth muscle, and c) myelin. The thyroid anitbodies are consistent with the histopathologic appearance of lymphocytic infiltration in her thyroid typical of autoimmune thyroiditis. Antibodies to smooth muscle are seen in chronic active hepatitis, but she had no clinical evidence of this. The clinical significance of antibodies to myelin has not yet been established, but the presence of such antibodies in a patient with myasthenia gravis is intriguing. No attempt was made to measure antibodies to acetylcholine receptors; however, most patients with myasthenia have been found to have such antibodies, and evidence suggests that such antibodies are, in fact, the cause of muscle weakness in this disease. Taken together, these findings indicate that the patient has an immunologic derangement resulting in the production of antibodies to multiple self-components, including thyroid, smooth muscle, myelin, and (probably) acetylcholine receptors. At least some of these antibodies appear to have resulted in pathologic changes in their target tissues resulting in the clinical symptoms of hypothyroidism and myasthenia gravis.

Hashimoto thyroiditis has been reported to occur frequently in cases of gonadal dysgenesis [34–41]. The finding of a high frequency of thyroid antibodies in such patients, as well as in their mothers, led to the suggestion that women with thyroid antibodies are predisposed to having children with chromosome aberrations [42–44]. One could incorporate the concept of genetic predisposition to the formation of autoantibodies into the following explanation: "The patient's mother and the patient both have a genetic tendency to form autoantibodies. The presence of antithyroid antibodies in the mother could predispose her to having a child with a chromosome aberration." However, we do not have such evidence in this kindred. Doniach and Roitt [45] also reported that the parents of their patients did not appear to have an increased incidence of higher antibody titers.

In addition to the possibility that autoimmunity induces chromosome defects, two other mechanisms could account for the association between autoimmunity and the Turner syndrome: 1) An X-chromosome defect could cause autoimmunity

[46–47]; 2) a common factor could underlie both autoimmunity and chromosomal accidents.

A relationship between the X chromosome and autoimmunity is supported by the following observations: A) The incidence of autoimmune diseases is higher in females than in males [48]; and B) congential agammaglobulinemia is an X-linked recessive condition and such patients frequently develop autoimmune conditions [49].

In view of the growing evidence that autoantibody formation is related to a deficiency in suppressor T cells which regulate B-cell differentiation and proliferation [50, 51], it is possible that the X chromosome contains genes that somehow influence suppressor T-cell differentiation, proliferation, or function. Of course other mechanisms [8, 52–54] could be postulated to account for these associations.

In summary, this extremely interesting association of lymphocytic thyroiditis and myasthenia gravis in a patient with Turner syndrome, hitherto undescribed, may be more than fortuitous. Patients with Turner syndrome having an abnormality of a sex chromosome may be particularly prone to develop thyroid autoantibodies and other concomitant autoimmune disorders.

ACKNOWLEDGMENT

We are indebted to Dr. Noel Rose for his helpful comments.

REFERENCES

1. Rose, NR, Witebsky E: Studies in organ specificity. V. Changes in the thyroid glands of rabbits following active immunization with rabbit thyroid extracts. J Immunol 76:417–427, 1956.
2. Witebsky E, Rose NR: Studies of organ specificity. IV. Production of rabbit thyroid antibodies in rabbit. J Immunol 76:408–416, 1956.
3. Roitt IM, Doniach D, Campbell PN, Hudson RV: Auto-antibodies in Hashimoto's disease (lymphadenoid goitre). Lancet 2:820–821, 1956.
4. Søborg M, Halberg P: Cellular hypersensitivity in Hashimoto's thyroiditis. Acta Med Scand 183:101–105, 1968.
5. Lamki L, Row VV, Volpé R: Cell-mediated immunity in Graves' disease and in Hashimoto's thyroiditis as shown by the demonstration of migration inhibition factor (MIF). J Clin Endocrinol Metab 36:358–364, 1973.
6. Simpson JA: Myasthenia gravis: A new hypothesis. Scott Med J 5:419–436, 1960.
7. Strauss AJL, Seegal BC, Hsu KC, Burkholder PM, Nastuk WL, Osserman KE: Immunofluorescence demonstration of a muscle-binding, complement-fixing serum globulin fraction in myasthenia gravis. Proc Soc Exp Biol Med 105:184–191, 1960.
8. Abdou NI, Lisak RP, Zweiman B, Abrahamsohn I, Penn AS: The thymus in myasthenia gravis: Evidence for altered cell populations. N Engl J Med 291:1271–1275, 1974.
9. Simpson JA, Behan PO, Dick HM: Studies on the nature of autoimmunity in myasthenia gravis: Evidence for an immunodeficiency type. Ann NY Acad Sci 274:382–389, 1976.
10. Grob D: Introduction: Myasthenia gravis in perspective. Ann NY Acad Sci 274:1–2, 1976.

11. Daly JJ, Jackon E: Case of Hashimoto's disease with myasthenia gravis. Br Med J 1:748, 1964.
12. Simpson JA: Immunological disturbances in myasthenia gravis with a report of Hashimoto's disease developing after thymectomy. J Neurol Neurosurg Psychiatry 27:485–492, 1964.
13. Singer W, Sahay BM: Myasthenia gravis, Hashimoto's thyroiditis, and pernicious anemia. Br Med J 1:904, 1966.
14. Osserman KE, Tsairis P, Weiner LB: Myasthenia gravis and thyroid disease: Clinical and immunologic correlation. J Mt Sinai Hosp 34:469–483, 1967.
15. Igata A, Takita K, Tsukagoshi H, Toyokura Y: A case of myasthenia gravis associated with Hashimoto's disease: With particular reference to the discrepancy between immunosuppressive effect of corticosteroids and myasthenia symptoms. Adv Neurol Sci (Tokyo) 14:471–475, 1970.
16. Sparagana M, Grieble H, Rubinstein H: Granulocytic leukemia associated with myxedema thyroiditis and myasthenia gravis. J Am Geriatr Soc 20:272–278, 1972.
17. Souadjian JV, Enriquez P, Silverstein MN, Pépin J-M: The spectrum of diseases associated with thymoma. Coincidence or syndrome? Arch Intern Med 134:374–379, 1974.
18. Osher RH, Smith JL: Ocular myasthenia gravis and Hashimoto's thyroiditis. Am J Ophthalmol 79:1038–1043, 1975.
19. Segal BM, Weintraub MI: Hashimoto's thyroiditis, myasthenia gravis, idiopathic thrombocytopenic purpura. Ann Intern Med 85:761–763, 1976.
20. Clagett JA, Wilson CB, Weigle WO: Interstitial immune complex thyroiditis in mice. The role of autoantibody to thyroglobulin. J Exp Med 140:1439–1456, 1974.
21. Appel SH, Almon RR, Levy N: Acetylcholine receptor antibodies in myasthenia gravis. N Engl J Med 293:760–761, 1975.
22. Bender AN, Ringel SP, Engel WK, Daniels MP, Vogel Z: Myasthenia gravis: A serum factor blocking acetylcholine receptors of the human neuromuscular junction. Lancet 1: 607–609, 1975.
23. Toyka KV, Drachman DB, Pestronk A, Kao I: Myasthenia gravis: Passive transfer from man to mouse. Science 190:397–399, 1975.
24. Engel AG, Lambert EH, Howard FM: Immune complexes (IgG and C_3) at the motor end-plate in myasthenia gravis. Mayo Clin Proc 52:267–280, 1977.
25. Pirskanen RA, Tiilikainen A, Hokkanen B: Histocompatability (HL-A) antigens associated with myasthenia gravis. Ann Clin Res 4:304–306, 1972.
26. Säfwenberg J, Lindblom JB, Osterman PO: HL-A frequencies in patients with myasthenia gravis. Tissue Antigens 3:465–469, 1973.
27. Behan PO, Simpson JA, Dick H: Immune response genes in myasthenia gravis. Lancet 2: 1033, 1973.
28. Feltkamp TEW, Van der Berg-Loonen PM, Nijenhuis LE, Engelfriet CP, Van Rossum AL, Van Loghem JJ, Oosterhuis HJGH: Myasthenia gravis, autoantibodies and HL-A antigens. Br Med J 1:131–133, 1974.
29. Fritze D, Herrmann C Jr, Naeim F, Smith GS, Walford RL: HL-A antigens in myasthenia gravis. Lancet 1:240–243, 1974.
30. Dick HM, Behan PO, Simpson JA, Durward WF: The inheritance of HL-A antigens in myasthenia gravis. J Immunogenet 1:401–412, 1974.
31. Fritze D, Herrmann C Jr, Naeim F, Smith GS, Eeller E, Walford RL: The biologic significance of HL-A antigen markers in myasthenia gravis. Ann NY Acad Sci 274:440–450, 1976.
32. Pirskanen R: On the significance of HL-A and LD antigens in myasthenia gravis. Ann NY Acad Sci 274:451–460, 1976.
33. Oosterhuis HJGH, Feltkamp TEW, Van Rossum AL, Van der Berg-Loonen PM, Nijenhuis LE: HL-A antigens, autoantibody production, and associated diseases in thymoma patients with and without myasthenia gravis. Ann NY Acad Sci 274:468–474, 1976.

34. Sparkes RS, Motulsky AG: Hashimoto's disease in Turner's syndrome with isochromosome X. Lancet 1:947, 1963.
35. Williams ED, Engel E, Forbes AP: Thyroiditis and gonadal dysgenesis. N Engl J Med 270: 805–810, 1964.
36. Grumbach MM, Morishima A: X-chromosome abnormalities in gonadal dysgenesis: DNA replication of structurally abnormal X-chromosomes; relation to thyroid disease (Abstract) J Pediatr 65:1087–1088, 1964.
37. Sparkes RS, Motulsky AG: The Turner syndrome with Isochromosome X and Hashimoto's thyroiditis. Ann Intern Med 67:132–144, 1967.
38. Hamilton CR, Moldawer M, Rosenberg HS: Hashimoto's thyroiditis and Turner's syndrome. Arch Intern Med 122:69–72, 1968.
39. Melin K, Samuelson G: Gonadal dysgenesis with lymphocytic thyroiditis and deletion of the long arm of the X chromosome. Acta Paediatr Scand 58:625–631, 1969.
40. Saito S, Sakurada T, Tayama S, Akihama T, Demura H, Demura R: A case of Turner's syndrome with juvenile Hashimoto's disease. Naika (Tokyo) 26:783–786, 1970.
41. Ouais SG, Trujillo J, Samaan NA: An atypical case of gonadal dysgenesis. Acta Endocrinol (Kbh) 70:365–372, 1972.
42. Fialkow PJ: Autoimmunity: A predisposing factor to chromosomal aberrations? Lancet 1:474–475, 1964.
43. Engel E, Forbes AP: Cytogenetic and clinical findings in 48 patients with congenitally defective or absent ovaries. Medicine 44:135–164, 1965.
44. Vallotton MB, Forbes AP: Autoimmunity in gonadal dysgenesis and Klinefelter's syndrome. Lancet 1:648–651, 1967.
45. Doniach D, Roitt IM, Polani PE: Thyroid antibodies and sex-chromosome anomalies. Proc R Soc Med 61:278–280, 1968.
46. Thompson H: Abnormalities of the autosomal chromosomes associated with human disease: Selected topics and catalogue. Am J Med Sci 250:718–734, 1965.
47. Williams ED, Engel E, Taft PD, Forbes AP: Gonadal dysgenesis and ulcerative colitis: A case report with clinical, cytogenetic, and postmortem studies. J Med Genet 3: 51–55, 1966.
48. Burch PRJ: Autoimmunity: Some aetiological aspects. Inflammatory polyarthritis and rheumatoid arthritis. Lancet 1:1253–1257, 1963.
49. Good RA, Kelly WD, Rotstein J, Varco RL: Immunological deficiency diseases, agammaglobulinemia, hypogammaglobulinemia, Hodgkin's disease and sarcoidosis. Prog Allergy 6:187–319, 1962.
50. Wick G, Sundick RS, Albini B: The obese strain (OS) of chickens: An animal model with spontaneous autoimmune thyroiditis. Clin Immunol Immunopathol 3:272–300, 1974.
51. Penhale WJ, Farmer A, Irvine WJ: Thyroiditis in T-cell depleted rats: Influence of strain, radiation dose, adjuvants and antilymphocyte serum. Clin Exp Immunol 21:362–375, 1975.
52. Weigle WO: Recent observations and concepts in immunological unresponsiveness and autoimmunity. Clin Exp Immunol 9:437–447, 1971.
53. Allison AC: Unresponsiveness to self-antigens. Lancet 2:1401–1403, 1971.
54. Simpson JA: Tolleranza immunologica e miastenia. Il vuolo deltimo nell'accrescimento e nella differenziazione. Riv Patol Nerv Ment 95:376–388, 1974.

SECTION III: TWIN STUDIES IN BIRTH DEFECT RESEARCH

Congenital Malformations: The Contribution of Twin Studies

Ntinos C. Myrianthopoulos, PhD

INTRODUCTION

Twin data in general and congenital malformations in particular are usually analyzed by making comparisons of concordance in monozygotic (MZ) and dizygotic (DZ) twins. These comparisons provide a very useful screening technique for dealing with conditions in which a genetic component is suspected, and for obtaining some measure of the relative importance of genetic and environmental factors. The underlying principle is simple: the members of a pair of MZ twins are genetically identical and permit observations of the effects of differing environments on the same genotype, while the members of a pair of DZ twins are genetically different and permit studies of the effects of similar environment on different genotypes. Thus, twin research is not so much a tool for genetic analysis as a means for testing hypotheses about environmental effects.

The practical application of this seemingly simple and elegant concept, however, is appreciably marred by several well-known experimental limitations and methodologic pitfalls [1], among which sampling bias and sufficient numbers must be placed at the top of the list. In the case of congenital malformations the twin method has the additional disadvantage of confusing shared genotype with shared egg cytoplasm.

There are, of course, other ways in which twin data can be informative, and I would like to present and discuss some aspects of congenital malformations which occurred in twins born in the Collaborative Perinatal Project.

The Collaborative Perinatal Project is a cooperative endeavor of 12 institutions throughout the United States and the National Institute of Neurological and Communicative Disorders and Stroke of the National Institutes of Health, to observe and study events which affect the parents before and during pregnancy and to relate them to the outcome of pregnancy. To this end, about 56,000 pregnant women have been followed from the first months of their pregnancy through labor and delivery, and the children born to Project mothers are being followed to the seventh year of life. The Project population is about 45% white, 47% black, 7% Puerto Rican, and the rest of a variety of other ethnic groups.

Birth Defects: Original Article Series, Volume XIV, Number 6A, pages 151–165

The collection of information, medical examinations, and laboratory tests have been done in uniform fashion and according to preestablished protocol.

Twin pregnancies, of course, constitute only a small fraction of all pregnancies, and even in a sizable population such as that of the Collaborative Perinatal Project the number of twins available for study of congenital malformations would not be as large as one would have desired. The advantages, however, of prospective selection, nearly complete ascertainment, frequent examinations in accordance with standardized protocol, and assessment of malformations with high accuracy make this a desirable twin population to study.

CRITERIA, DEFINITIONS, AND MATERIALS

The criteria for selection and definitions of congenital malformations have been described in detail in previous reports on malformations in singletons [2] and in twins [3]. Briefly, a congenital malformation is defined as a gross physical or anatomic developmental anomaly which was present at birth or was detected during the first year of life. Malformations were divided into major and minor with some degree of arbitrariness: a malformation is considered major if it affects the individual adversely by causing increased mortality and morbidity. Otherwise it is considered minor.

The epidemiologic characteristics of twins born in the Collaborative Perinatal Project were described in a previous publication [4]. To summarize, 615 pairs of twins were born among 56,249 pregnancies with known outcome, or 1 in 91.5 births. Among whites there were 259 twin births in 25,991 pregnancies, or 1 in 100.3 births; among blacks there were 331 twin births in 26,080 pregnancies, or 1 in 78.8 births; and among the Other group, consisting of Puerto Rican, there were 25 twin births in 4,178 pregnancies, or 1 in 167.1 births.

The zygosity of 508 pairs of twins was established by comparison of sex, nine blood group systems (ABO, MNS, Rh, P, Kell, Lewis, Lutheran, Duffy, and Kidd), and gross and microscopic examination of the placenta. In 118 pairs the zygosity could not be determined. In some of these pairs one or both twins died early, before zygosity tests could be done, and placental examinations were not available or were inconclusive. Some were lost to the Project either because they were born outside a Project hospital or because their families withdrew their cooperation, and in a few, the sex of one or both twins could not be determined.

Among white twins 34.6% were monozygotic and 65.4% dizygotic; among black twins 28.8% were MZ and 71.2% DZ; and among twins in the Other group, 60.0% were MZ and 40.0% DZ.

Included in this study are 1,197 twin individuals for whom information about the presence or absence of malformations was available. Their distribution by zygosity and completeness of pairs is shown in Table 1. This number includes

TABLE 1. Twins at Risk for Malformations

	Complete pairs	Incomplete pairs	Individuals
Monozygotic	187	1	375
Dizygotic	308	1	617
Zygosity undetermined	87	31	205
Total	582	33	1,197

115 fetal and neonatal deaths for whom clinical and autopsy findings were available. Pairs were considered complete if information concerning malformations was available for both members of a pair whether the twins were alive or dead. As is evident from Table 1, most of the incomplete pairs were in the zygosity undetermined (ZU) category.

Also included in this count is a pair of stillborn thoracopagus monozygotic female twins with multiple cardiovascular, alimentary, and other malformations. Because of the rarity and uniqueness of conjoined twinning, and the difficulty in ascribing the overall malformation as well as the specific malformations to one or the other twin, this pair was excluded from the calculation of malformation frequencies. It is used, however, in subsequent special analyses.

RESULTS

Malformations in Twins and Singletons

Table 2 shows the distribution of malformations in twins by zygosity. The last column gives the distribution of malformations in singletons from the same population for comparison. Numbers in parentheses represent frequencies of multiple malformations and individuals with multiple malformations; frequencies for single malformations are obtained by simple subtraction. Among 1,195 twin individuals for whom information about malformations was available, 219 or 18.33% were born with malformations – 179 or 14.98% with single and 40 or 3.35% with multiple malformations. The total number of malformations was 294, of which 115 were multiple and were counted as many times as they occurred in an individual. Among malformed twins, 18.26% had more than one malformation, and 39.12% of malformations were associated with some other malformation.

Table 2 also shows that the frequency of malformations and malformed individuals is higher in twins than in singletons. Among 53,257 single deliveries

TABLE 2. Distribution of Malformations in Twins by Zygosity, and in Singletons*

	Twins				
	Monozygotic	Dizygotic	Zygosity undetermined	Total	Singletons
Total number of malformations	119 (44)	112 (36)	63 (35)	294 (115)	10,480 (3,574)
Total number of malformed cases	90 (15)	91 (15)	38 (10)	219 (40)	8,288 (1,382)
Total number of individuals	373	617	205	1,195	53,257
Frequency (mean number) of malformations	0.319	0.181	0.307	0.246	0.197
Frequency of malformed cases (%)	24.13 (4.02)	14.75 (2.43)	18.54 (4.88)	18.33 (3.35)	15.56 (2.59)
Frequency of multiple malformations among all malformations (%)	36.97	32.14	55.56	39.12	34.10
Frequency of mutiple malformed cases among all malformed cases (%)	16.67	16.48	26.32	18.26	16.67

*Numbers in parentheses are multiple malformations.

in the Collaborative Perinatal Project, 8,288 or 15.56% were born with malformations – 6,906 or 12.97% with single and 1,382 or 2.59% with multiple malformations. The increase of malformed twins over singletons is significant (χ_1^2 = 6.76). Among malformed singletons 16.67% had more than one malformation, and 34.10% of malformations were associated with some other malformation. The increase, however, of multiple malformations and multiply malformed individuals in twins over singletons is not significant.

These are among the highest malformation rates reported for twins and singletons. The high frequency of malformations could easily be explained on the basis of the period of time through which the malformations were observed and the conditions which made almost complete ascertainment possible.

It becomes evident, from closer inspection of Table 2, that the difference is solely contributed by an increase of malformations in MZ twins that is highly significant (χ_1^2 = 20.62). DZ twins, if anything, show a slight decrease in frequency of malformations compared to singletons, but this is not significant. ZU twins show a frequency intermediate between those of MZ and DZ twins and similar to the overall twin malformation frequency. This is understandable since ZU twins compromise a mixture of MZ and DZ like-sexed twins.

The increase in frequency of malformations in MZ twins holds true for both major and minor malformations, as seen in Table 3. The frequency of malformed MZ twins is significantly increased over that of singletons in all three malformation categories – *major only, major and minor,* and *minor only* (χ_1^2 = 7.35, 4.59, and 7.39, respectively), while the frequency of DZ twins is about the same in the *major only,* and *major and minor* categories, and substantially decreased in the *minor only* category. Twins of unknown zygosity have the highest frequency in the *major only* category and the lowest in the *minor only* category. This is not surprising, for most twins of unknown zygosity are fetal deaths and have a high rate of major malformations which are probably the cause of death.

Malformations by System

Table 4 gives the distribution of malformations by system or type in twins and singletons. Most frequent overall are malformations of the musculoskeletal system, followed by malformations of the alimentary tract, skin, and ear. Less frequent and of about the same proportions are malformations of the cardiovascular, upper respiratory, central nervous and genitourinary systems.

The most impressive feature of the comparison is the significant more than twofold increase in twins of cardiovascular and alimentary tract malformations. Less impressive was the degree of central nervous system and related skeletal malformations, though the difference for this system is not significant. These are practically all major malformations. Significantly increased are also ear malfor-

TABLE 3. Distribution of Twins and Singletons by Major and Minor Malformations, and Percentages

	Twins				
	MZ	DZ	ZU	Total	Singletons
Major	40 10.72	48 7.78	25 12.20	113 9.46	3,781 7.10
Major and minor	9 2.41	9 1.46	4 1.95	22 1.84	641 1.20
Minor	41 10.99	34 5.51	9 4.39	84 7.03	3,866 7.26
Total number of individuals	373	617	205	1,195	53,257

TABLE 4. Frequency of Malformations by System in Twins and Singletons

	Twins		Singletons	
System or type	Rate per 1,000	% of malformations	Rate per 1,000	% of malformations
Central nervous system and related skeletal	15.07	6.12	10.31	5.24
Musculoskeletal	51.88	21.09	52.54	26.70
Eye	5.02	2.04	4.07	2.07
Ear	26.78	10.89	18.02	9.16*
Upper respiratory tract and mouth	15.90	6.46	11.23	5.71
Thoracic	6.69	2.72	4.77	2.42
Cardiovascular	17.57	7.14	7.57	3.85***
Alimentary tract	42.68	17.35	19.32	9.82***
Liver, bile, and spleen	5.02	2.04	0.51	0.25***
Genitourinary	12.55	5.10	16.56	8.42
Tumors	0.00	0.00	0.66	0.33
Skin	45.19	18.37	48.48	24.64
Syndromes	1.67	0.68	1.99	1.01
Endocrine and metabolic	0.00	0.00	0.47	0.24
Infection	0.00	0.00	0.28	0.14
Total		100.00		100.00

$^*P \leqslant 0.05$; $^{***}P \leqslant 0.001$.

mations and malformations of the upper respiratory tract and mouth, which comprise a mixture of major and minor malformations. Genitourinary and skin malformations, on the other hand, are slightly decreased in twins.

Malformations in Live Births and Fetal and Later Deaths

Table 5 gives the frequencies of malformations in twins and singletons who survived to one year, fetal and neonatal deaths, and those who died from 28 days to one year. It is evident that the significant increase of malformations in twins over singletons occurred only in live births who survived to one year. In fact, among all deaths singletons have a higher frequency of malformations than twins but the difference is not significant. The small increases of malformations in twin fetal deaths and in deaths that occurred from 28 days to one year are not significant. On the other hand, among neonatal deaths singletons have a significantly higher frequency of malformations than twins ($\chi_1^2 = 4.32$).

Race and Sex Differences

Table 6 shows the frequency of twins with malformations by race and sex, compared with that of singletons. Black twins show a slight but significant increase in malformations over white twins ($\chi_1^2 = 4.46$) but, as in the case of singletons, the difference is almost entirely due to a higher frequency in blacks of the minor malformations, polydactyly and branchial cleft anomalies. However, the proportion of malformed black twins is much higher than that of black singletons when compared to white twins and singletons. The increase in malformation frequency in the Other group is intermediate between those of whites and blacks, but the number of Other twin pairs is quite small and subject to sampling error. There is no difference in major or multiple malformations between white and black twins.

Male twins are more frequently malformed than female, following the pattern of singletons, but the difference is not significant.

Male twins show a significant increase in malformations over male singletons ($\chi_1^2 = 4.55$), while the increase in female twins is slight and not significant. It is interesting to note that the increase in malformation frequency in male over female twins is about the same as that of male over female singletons.

There is a slight overall increase in multiple malformations in twins over singletons but this is not significant and agrees with previous observations. When examined by race and sex, however, the distribution shows some interesting differences. There is a small and about equal increase in multiple malformations in white and black twins over singletons, but a decrease in the Other group. It is evident that the increase, which is significant ($\chi_1^2 = 5.28$), is totally contributed by female twins.

TABLE 5. Malformations in Live Births, Surviving to One Year, and in Fetal and Neonatal Deaths, and in Deaths up to One Year in Twins and Singletons

	Twins			Singletons		
	No. of individuals	No. of malformations	% of malformations	No. of individuals	No. of malformations	% of malformations
Live births – surviving to one year	995	186	18.69	51,096	7,856	15.37
Fetal deaths	74	7	9.46	1,004	82	8.17
Neonatal deaths	108	21	19.44	877	255	29.08
Deaths from 28 days to one year	18	5	27.78	417	98	23.50
Total deaths	200	33	16.50	2,298	435	18.93

TABLE 6. Frequency of Twins With Malformations Compared With That of Singletons, by Race and Sex (%)

	Twins		Singletons	
	With at least one malformation	With multiple malformations	With at least one malformation	With multiple malformations
White	15.69	3.42	14.73	2.60
Black	20.59	3.43	16.80	2.63
Other	15.79	1.75	12.79	2.29
Male	20.37	3.03	17.03	3.17
Female	16.31	3.66	14.04	1.99
Total	18.33	3.35	15.56	2.59

Concordance of Twins for Malformations

It is altogether remarkable that congenital malformations should be increased only in MZ twins, yet in itself, MZ twinning can be considered a congenital malformation. The cause of such increase, and of MZ twinning for that matter, is unknown. It is tempting and reasonable to speculate that a common mechanism may be responsible for both MZ twinning and congenital malformations, but there is no evidence for this, at least in man. It might be instructive to examine the occurrence of malformations in co-twins and the concordance rate of MZ and DZ twins, bearing in mind the limitations and pitfalls of this approach, mentioned earlier. The important and catastrophic malformations, of course, are also very rare, so that even in a relatively large sample of twins there is not a sufficient number of them for comparison. The number of useful and informative comparisons is reduced even further because these can be made only in unbroken pairs of known zygosity. The comparisons, therefore, have to be confined to major categories of malformations.

Table 7 shows that the concordance rate of MZ twins is consistently and significantly higher than that of DZ twins in all comparison categories. The difference in major malformations, though significant, is not as large as would be expected. This is not surprising, for most of the major catastrophic malformations occurred in broken pairs of unknown zygosity, which were necessarily eliminated from the comparison. The impressive fact is that in a significant number of cases when one twin of a pair had a malformation, the co-twin also had a malformation though not necessarily the same as that of the first twin. Among 23 pairs of MZ twins concordant for any malformation, 16 or 69% were concordant for at least one similar malformation while 7 or 30.4% were concordant for different

TABLE 7. Concordance and Discordance of Twins for Malformations†

Malformation		Concordance	Discordance	Concordance rate	χ_1^2
Any malformation	MZ	23	46	0.34	16.52***
	DZ	6	79	0.07	
Major	MZ	9	20	0.31	4.16*
	DZ	4	39	0.09	
Minor	MZ	7	30	0.23	3.97*
	DZ	1	31	0.03	
Major and minor	MZ	7	3	0.70	5.21*
	DZ	1	9	0.10	
Single	MZ	16	40	0.29	8.17**
	DZ	5	62	0.07	
Multiple	MZ	4	33	0.12	6.48*
	DZ	0	86	0.00	
Single or multiple	MZ	23	29	0.44	9.18**
	DZ	6	38	0.14	

†Includes the pair of conjoined twins. *$P \leqslant 0.05$; **$P \leqslant 0.01$; ***$P \leqslant 0.001$.

malformations. All 6 concordant DZ twins, however, were concordant for at least one similar malformation. Even so, when MZ and DZ twins concordant for the same malformation are compared, the concordance rate of MZ is still significantly higher ($\chi_1^2 = 6.82$).

Though genetic factors play some role in the occurrence of malformations in twins, they cannot account for the increase of malformations in MZ twins over DZ twins and singletons, for the probability of occurrence of genetic malformations should be equal in MZ and DZ twins. Therefore, the excess malformations in MZ twins must be due to environmental factors, either acting directly on the developing embryo, or interacting with the genetic determinants for normal embryonic development.

The Role of the Placenta

The importance of the human placenta in such processes is obvious. It is a physical and physiologic link between mother and fetus, and exhibits variations with regard to membrane type, size, and circulation that may be important in themselves or may affect the nutrition of the embryo or the transport of drugs, toxins, and infectious agents, which are important in the production of malformations.

The placentation of DZ twins is the same as that of singletons – each DZ twin individual is surrounded by a separate amnion and a separate chorion. MZ twins, however, can be either monochorionic (MC) or dichorionic (DC) depending on the time of separation of the cell mass which results in the two embryos. Since DZ twins have the same placentation and the same malformation rate as singletons, we will confine our attention to differences in the placentation of MZ twins.

Several studies have shown that about two-thirds of MZ twins are MC and one-third DC [5]. Our data, shown in Table 8, agree with these figures. Among the 188 MZ pairs, 117 were MC and 56 DC, giving a ratio of 2.09:1. In 15 pairs the placentation could not be determined either because the placental material was unsuitable for examination or because the examination was not conclusive.

Now, if we hypothesize that the excess malformations are environmentally induced and due to influences of placental type or circulation, then we would expect higher proportions of malformations in MC than in DC twins. The data in Table 8 do not support this hypothesis. The distribution by placental type of pairs with malformations is not significantly different from that of all pairs, and the frequency of MC pairs with malformations is not significantly different from that of DC pairs. The same is true when twins are considered as individuals rather than in pairs (Table 9). MC and DC MZ twins have frequencies of malformations in proportion to their distribution in the general population.

Concordance studies with regard to placental type should be illuminating, but with comparisons restricted to MZ pairs only, the available small numbers become even smaller. The findings, therefore, must be interpreted with caution.

Among the 66 pairs with one or both members malformed, the placental type was known in 59 pairs (42 MC and 17 DC); in 7 pairs the placental type was not known. Under the previously mentioned hypothesis we would expect significantly higher concordance among MC than among DC twins. It is evident from Table 10 that this is not the case. If anything, the concordance rate is higher among DC than among MC twins. This finding may be due to sampling error because of the small number of DC pairs. The binomial probability of obtaining this placental distribution of concordant pairs under the 1:1 hypothesis is 0.168. These data, again, lend no support to the hypothesis of placental effects.

Table 11 describes the malformations for which the 23 MZ pairs were concordant. Notice that not all of them were concordant for the same malformation. Sixteen pairs, or 69.6%, were concordant for at least one similar malformation and seven pairs, or 30.4%, were concordant for different malformations. Two pairs (Nos. 12 and 22) were MA-MC. The former is the pair of conjoined thoracopagus twins mentioned earlier. This pair has been described in detail elsewhere because of some interesting events in the history of the mother before and during pregnancy [3, 6].

TABLE 8. Distribution of All MZ Pairs and Pairs With Malformations, by Placental Type

Placenta	All pairs	Pairs with malformations	% pairs with malformations
Monochorionic (MC)	117	42	35.90
Dichorionic (DC)	56	17	30.36
Unknown	15	7	46.67
Total	188	66	35.11
MC/DC ratio	2.09:1	2.47:1	

TABLE 9. Distribution of Malformed Individuals in MZ Pairs With Malformations

Placenta	Pairs $\times$ 2	Malformed individuals	% malformed individuals
Monochorionic (MC)	84	58	69.05
Dichorionic (DC)	34	24	70.59
Unknown	14	10	71.43
Total	132	92	69.70

TABLE 10. Concordance and Discordance of MC and DC MZ Twins in Malformed Sample

Placenta	Concordance	Discordance	Concordance rate
Monochorionic (MC)	11	31	0.26
Dichorionic (DC)	10	7	0.59
Unknown	2	5	0.26

$\chi_1^2 = 4.29$, $P < 0.05$.

TABLE 11. Malformations in Concordant MZ Twins

	Placenta[a]	Twin A	Twin B
1	DC	Undescended testis	Undescended testis
2	MC	Macrocephaly	Hydrocephaly
3	DC	Metatarsus adductus; undescended testis	Metatarsus adductus
4	MC	Metatarsus adductus	Metatarsus adductus
5	DC	Metatarsus adductus	Metatarsus adductus
6	DC	Clinodactyly	Clinodactyly
7	DC	Preauricular sinus	Ventricular septal defect
8	DC	Cystic kidney	Cardiac enlargement
9	MC	Focal malformation of bile duct; cystic kidney	Focal malformation of bile duct
10	MC	Hyperflexibility of knee joints	Anencephaly; cleft lip and palate; cor triloculare; absence of gallbladder; vertebral abnormality
11	DC	Polydactyly	Polydactyly
12	MC	Conjoined thoracopagus twins with fused hearts, livers, common umbilical cord, and single placenta	
13	MC	Tracheoesophageal fistula	Cardiac enlargement; strawberry hemangioma
14	MC	Polydactyly	Polydactyly
15	DC	Deformed ear pinna	Deformed ear pinna
16	Unk	Metatarsus adductus; inguinal hernia	Metatarsus adductus
17	MC	Metatarsus adductus	Metatarsus adductus
18	MC	Metatarsus adductus	Preauricular sinus
19	Unk	Talipes equinovarus	Metatarsus adductus
20	DC	Deformed ear pinna; talipes calcaneovalgus	Deformed ear pinna; fibrous dysplasia of bone
21	DC	Pyloric stenosis; umbilical hernia; inguinal hernia	Pyloric stenosis; umbilical hernia; inguinal hernia
22	MC	Supernumerary nipples; café-au-lait spots	Supernumerary nipples; café-au-lait spots
23	MC	Preauricular skin tag	Preauricular skin tag

[a] DC – dichorionic; MC – monochorionic; Unk – unknown.

Some of these malformations are known to be genetic in origin (polydactyly, clinodactyly, supernumerary nipples, pyloric stenosis). Even when pairs with these genetic malformations are excluded (Table 12), the distribution of placental types does not appreciably change – 9 pairs are MC and 7 DC. The binomial probability of obtaining this distribution under the 1:1 hypothesis is 0.175.

These findings, though based on small numbers, provide fairly convincing evidence that the placenta and placental circulation per se do not contribute to the excess of malformations seen in MZ twins.

TABLE 12. Placental Type of Concordant MZ Twins

Placenta	All pairs	Excluding pairs with genetic malformations[a]
Monochorionic (MC)	11	9
Dichorionic (DC)	10	7
Unknown	2	2

[a]Clinodactyly, # 6; polydactyly, # 11, 14; pyloric stenosis, # 21; supernumerary nipples, # 22.

A NEW HYPOTHESIS

I wish at this point to propose a new hypothesis, developed in collaboration with Dr. Michael Melnick, that the excess of malformations in MZ twins is the result of a two-hit process: 1) The MZ twinning process which may occur anywhere from the premorula to the blastula stage disrupts the developmental genetic clock of the embryo; and 2) this disruption effects numerical and temporal biochemical disadvantages in the two resulting embryos and renders them susceptible to the action of subtle environmental agents.

It is conceivable that the disadvantages of cell number and possibly biochemical timing which are brought about by the twinning process are in themselves sufficiently severe to increase significantly the malformation frequency in MZ twins. We consider it more likely, however, that the increase in malformations is due to the synergistic action of a disadvantaged embryo and exposure to environmental agents that would be either nonteratogenic or only mildly teratogenic in DZ twins and in singletons who had not been subjected to the first hit. The list of such agents in our world of increasing industrial and pharmacologic pollution is certainly on the rise. To test this hypothesis, a study using Collaborative Perinatal Project data is presently under way to analyze epidemiologically the frequency of drug intake, viral infections, febrile episodes, etc, during pregnancy of mothers of MZ twins in comparison to that of mothers of DZ twins and singletons.

Approaches of this sort may not only provide an explanation for the increased frequency of malformations in MZ twins but may also enhance our still lamentably meager understanding of the interaction between genes and environment in common disorders of man.

REFERENCES

1. Allen G: Twin research: Problems and prospects. In Steinberg AG, Bearn AG (eds): "Progress in Medical Genetics." New York: Grune & Stratton, 1965, vol 4, pp 242–269.
2. Myrianthopoulos NC, Chung CS: "Congenital Malformations in Singletons: Epidemiologic Survey." Miami: Symposia Specialists for The National Foundation–March of Dimes. BD:OAS X (11):1974.
3. Myrianthopoulos NC: "Congenital Malformations in Twins: Epidemiologic Survey." Miami: Symposia Specialists for The National Foundation–March of Dimes. BD:OAS XI(8): 1975.
4. Myrianthopoulos NC: An epidemiologic survey of twins in a large, prospectively studied population. Am J Hum Genet 22:611–629, 1970.
5. Bulmer MG: "The Biology of Twinning in Man." Oxford: Clarendon Press, 1970.
6. Myrianthopoulos NC, Burdé B: A case of conjoined twins. Acta Genet Med Gemellol (Roma) 25:59–61, 1976.

The Use of Twin Registers in the Study of Birth Defects*

Joe C. Christian, PhD, MD

INTRODUCTION

Twins have long been favorite subjects for students of human development. Studies have ranged from surveys of large twin registers to reports based on a single twin pair. Twins provide pairs of individuals of the same age and from similar environments who may be genetically identical (monozygotic, or MZ) pairs, or who may be no more genetically similar than sibs born of different pregnancies (dizygotic, or DZ).

There is increasing evidence that twins are subject to unique stresses by the twinning process itself. For example twins, in particular MZ twins, have a greater incidence of certain congenital anomalies than singletons [1, 2]. This paper will explore the possibilities of making use, to further exploit the relationships of twins in the study of human development, of twin registers (the terms register and registry are often used synonymously [3], in this paper register will be used throughout). In particular, evidence will be reviewed that indicates how studies of associations between developmental parameters and type of twin may provide clues as to the etiology of birth defects.

ASSOCIATION OF TWINS AND QUANTITATIVE VARIABLES

Many traits of interest in human development vary along a continuous scale of values and are called quantitative or metric characters. Their study depends upon measurement rather than upon tabulating whether the trait is present or absent. It is possible for the mean, variance, skewness, or kurtosis of a quantita-

*This article is publication No 77-31 from the Department of Medical Genetics and was supported in part by the Indiana University Human Genetics Center, PHS GM 21054, NIH contract No 71-2307 and a grant from the John A. Hartford Foundation, Inc.

Birth Defects: Original Article Series, Volume XIV, Number 6A, pages 167–178

tive trait to be associated with twinning. However, in practice only the mean and variance are usually considered.

The test to determine if there is an association between type of twin and the mean of a quantitative trait is often not done on twin data, and when it is done, an independent-samples t test is usually applied and usually incorrectly applied. The independent-samples t test treats the twins in MZ and DZ pairs – examples of the closest of human genetic and environmental relationships – as if they were independent individuals. Data collected from a series of pairs of MZ and DZ twins in reality have a nested structure: Pairs are nested within zygosities and individuals are nested within pairs. Zygosity is a fixed effect being set at or shortly after conception. Twin pairs, nested within zygosities, constitute a random effect. Finally, individuals nested within the twin pairs are another random effect. Statisticians label this structure a mixed-model (a mixture of random and fixed effects) nested design [4]. As a result of this structure, taking recognition of the fact that the expected values of the mean square among DZ pairs and among MZ pairs are not equal [5], the appropriate test of the difference between the means of MZ and DZ twins becomes an approximate t' test [6]. Similar tests may be used to test the difference between the means of twins and singletons and between subtypes of MZ twins.

There are little data on association of mean values of quantitative traits with type of twins. However, Havlik et al [7] recently reported that 4 of 11 clinical chemistry values provided evidence for unequal means of MZ and DZ twins ($P < 0.05$) in 514 pairs of adult male twins from the National Heart, Lung and Blood Institute (NHLBI) Collaborative Twin Study. The association of a twin type and the means of quantitative traits may therefore be relatively common and certainly should be searched for.

The association of twin type with the variance of a quantitative trait may be tested by comparing the sum of the mean squares within and among DZ pairs with the corresponding sum for MZ pairs by an F' test [5]. In the NHLBI twin study, 15 of 31 quantitative variables were found to have unequal total variances of MZ and DZ twins ($P < 0.05$) [8]. In addition, Reed et al [9] reported that 21 of 71 dermatoglyphic variables had unequal total variances of MZ and DZ twins. The association of twin type with the variance of quantitative traits, as with the mean, does not appear, therefore, to be unusual. The F' test on the total variance is a relatively insensitive test, however, and large numbers of twins are generally necessary to detect a difference between the total variances of MZ and DZ twins.

As an example of how association of variance with type of twinning may be used to gain insight into the etiology of that variation, the twin analyses of variance for right thumb and index finger ridge counts from the publication of Reed et al [9] are compared (Table 1). These variables were chosen as examples because they indicate different sources of variation for adjacent digit ridge counts, which are generally lumped into total ridge count. Total ridge count is

TABLE 1. Twin Analysis of Variance for Right Thumb and Index Finger Ridge Counts [9]

		Right thumb			Right index finger		
	n	MS_A	MS_W	Sum	MS_A	MS_W	Sum
MZ pairs	260	47.8	5.6	53.4	78.4	7.3	85.7
DZ pairs	163	63.0	23.2	86.2	61.3	32.9	94.2

n = number of twin pairs; MS_A = mean square among twin pairs; MS_W = mean square within twin pairs; Sum = $MS_A + MS_W$.

often used as an example of a trait influenced by multiple factors, the majority of which are assumed to be genetic [10].

For the right thumb ridge count, the sum of the MZ mean squares was found to be significantly smaller than the DZ sum ($P < 0.01$). The smaller total variance of MZ twins was interpreted to be due to a difference in environmental variance components for the two types of twins for this variable [9]. Because ridge counts are fixed long before birth, it therefore seemed reasonable to search for prenatal environmental influences that are different for MZ and DZ twins. A series of MZ twins of known placental type were studied and the within-dichorionic MZ-pair mean square was found to be significantly smaller than the within-monochorionic MZ-pair mean square for thumb ridge count [11]. This difference in mean squares is consistent with the smaller total variance for thumb ridge count in MZ twins of unknown placental type, compared to DZ twins, because approximately one-third of all MZ twins are dichorionic [12]. The comparison of within-pair mean squares between the two types of MZ twins is a valid test for a difference in the environmental variance components in the two types of MZ twins because neither mean square contains a genetic component of variance. This is in contrast to a comparison of within-pair mean squares of MZ and DZ pairs which may involve both genetic and environmental variance components [5]. Ridge count of the index finger, in contrast, revealed neither evidence for unequal total variances of MZ and DZ twins nor unequal within-pair mean squares of monochorionic-MZ and dichorionic-MZ pairs. The ridge development of the thumb, therefore, appears to be influenced more by prenatal environment, at least in twins, than ridge development of the index finger. In addition to ridge counts, variation of other dermatoglyphic variables has been shown to be associated with placental type. Noteworthy are the measures of placement of the palmar acial triradius, including *atd* angle, which have greater variability within monochorionic-MZ than within dichorionic-MZ pairs [11]. Associations of placental type and within-pair variance of MZ twins have also been found for hematocrit [13], IgG [14], plasma cholesterol [15], birthweight [16], and IQ [17].

QUALITATIVE TRAITS

In contrast to quantitative traits which are measured, qualitative traits, in the strictest sense, are either present or absent. The dividing line between qualitative and quantitative traits is not always clear but for this discussion, a qualitative trait will refer to the presence or absence of a developmental anomaly. Epidemiologic data about qualitative traits therefore will consist of counts of individuals with and without the defect in question. Twin pairs may be of three types for a single qualitative trait – both twins normal, one affected, or both affected. Twin analysis of qualitative traits and concordance rates requires modification of the methods for quantitative traits and has been previously reviewed [18, 19].

The test for association of the "mean" with twin type becomes, for qualitative data, a test for differences in the relative frequency of affected individuals between populations of twins and singletons or between different types of twins. The comparison of within-pair mean squares for MZ and DZ twins may be compared to a test of the difference between concordance rates of twin types.

Frequencies of a number of congenital anomalies have been found to be increased in MZ twins, but little is known about the relative frequencies of these anomalies in monochorionic- and dichorionic-MZ twins or the differences in concordance rates for these twin types. In data from the Collaborative Perinatal Project, Myrianthopoulos and Melnick [20] found no significant difference in the frequency of total malformations in monochorionic-MZ and dichorionic-MZ twins. These authors did find a significantly greater concordance rate for dichorionic-MZ twins than monochorionic-MZ twins, when all congenital anomalies were considered together. Acardia is an extreme example of a developmental anomaly that in man occurs only in discordant monochorionic-MZ pairs [21]. In all probability there are less extreme examples of associations between placental type of MZ pairs and developmental variables.

Smith, Bartlett, and Harrah [22] postulated that the association of MZ twinning and the Duhamel anomalad (imperforate anus to sirenomelia) was due to similar defects in embryonic center or disk development that result in MZ twinning and the Duhamel anomalad. Nance [23] and Giroud [24] suggested that discordance of MZ twins for anomalies such as anencephaly and sirenomelia could be due to segregation of cytoplasmic factors when the twins divided. Opitz, Summitt, and Smith [25] and Summitt and Wilroy [26] observed an apparent increase in the frequency of affected twins as well as unaffected twins in the relatives of patients with the hypertelorism-hypospadias syndrome and concluded that possibly the genetic defect causing this syndrome, apparently a single mutant gene, also predisposes the embryo to form MZ twins. It would be of interest to search for associations between placental type and all of these anomalies. For example, finding an association with MZ twinning and an association with a specific placental type of MZ twin, in contrast to finding association with MZ twinning but no association with placental type, could indicate different causes for the associations.

An imaginative approach that may also be applicable to association studies is that of Ross and Coupes [27], who combined quantitative and qualitative traits by studying craniofacial morphology in the unaffected co-twins of MZ pairs discordant for cleft lip and palate.

NEEDS AND AVAILABLE RESOURCES

In order to pursue studies of associations between relatively rare developmental anomalies and twinning, large populations must be surveyed to provide sufficient numbers to obtain meaningful results. In addition to detailed examination for developmental anomalies, accurate zygosity typing and placental examinations are also needed. Accurate zygosity determination is important in the study of the relationships between congenital anomalies and twinning for two reasons. First, it is important to distinguish like-sex MZ and DZ twin pairs. Second, in the comparisons of dichorionic-MZ and monochorionic-MZ twins, it becomes extremely important to have as few errors as possible in zygosity assignment, because most errors will result in DZ twins being labeled dichorionic MZ twins. These errors, if common enough, could either obscure associations with placental type or cause associations with zygosity to be ascribed to MZ placental type. Zygosity determination may be done by combinations of questionnaires, physical findings, and genetic markers. Genetic markers are the most precise, and with the large number of marker systems presently available, including red cell antigens, protein polymorphisms, and other systems such as HLA, the limiting factor usually becomes one of financial resources. One means of zygosity discrimination that perhaps will become more important is the study of inherited chromosome polymorphisms [28]. In particular, if karyotyping is being done for other reasons, this information should not be overlooked in determining zygosity.

Placental typing is critical for comparisons of MZ subtypes. Examination of the placenta should include gross and microscopic examination and, if there is interest in details of vascular anastomoses within the monochorionic-MZ pairs, examination should also be done following injection of the blood vessels. Unfortunately, in practice twin placentas are often discarded before any detailed examination is done.

There are a large number of subdivisions of MZ twins that might be important in association studies. Monochorionic-MZ twins can be further subdivided into mono- and diamnionic pairs and according to whether or not anastomoses are present between the fetal circulations. If anastomoses are present, their degree and type may also be recorded. Dichorionic-MZ twins may be further subdivided into those with fused or separate placentas, and relative placental size recorded. Other subdivisions that may be important are whether or not the twins are mirror images and, of course, if they are conjoined twins. Information may also be gained by looking for interaction of twin type and sex of the twins. The possibilities for association studies are therefore almost endless.

In 1965 the World Health Organization held a meeting of investigators interested in using twin registers for research. The conclusions from this meeting were subsequently published [29] and remain today an excellent review of the use of twins in epidemiologic studies such as the association of twin type with abnormal development. At the same time an international survey was made of active twin registers and studies [30]. Table 2 is a 1977 tabulation of twin registers in the United States and Canada, with the registers arranged alphabetically by states. In addition to the registers listed in Table 2 there are a number of other centers equipped to help with twin studies, in particular with zygosity diagnosis. These centers are listed in the International Directory of Genetic Services [31]. There are also over 400 Mothers of Twins Clubs in the United States and Canada eager to provide twins for research. The International Society for Twin Studies is also an excellent source of information on twin studies [32] and has a series of working groups designed to assist investigators.

The twin resources listed in Table 2, extensive as they are, are not adequate for detailed studies of associations between developmental anomalies and twin type. The twin panel from the Collaborative Perinatal Project [33] does, however, provide a model for future studies, and investigators actively involved in the other studies listed are an invaluable source of expertise.

The most acute need for association studies appears to be accurate and detailed placental examinations. As twin births are relatively rare and high-risk events, perhaps a case could be made for examination of all twin placentas. Certainly detailed placental examination is critical for any twins that later will be used in research.

SUMMARY

The study of associations between twin type and developmental anomalies is presented as a unique informative method of studying the etiology of abnormal development. Detailed study of the association of twinning and development will require large numbers of twins of known zygosity and placental type that are hopefully ascertained with minimal bias.

TABLE 2. Twin Studies and Registers in Canada and the United States in 1977

Register	Purpose of research	Data recorded and source of twins	Total number of twin pairs	Remarks
Canada				
1. McMaster University Twin Registry Irene Uchida, PhD Dept. of Pediatrics McMaster University Medical Centre 1200 Main Street Hamilton, Ontario Canada L8S 4J9 Ph: (416) 525-9140 Extension 2739/50	Study placental effects on traits in adult twins.	Placental data and birth records of twins born in Toronto from 1936 to 1959. Zygosity determination by genetic markers.	1,742	Perhaps the only adult twin panel on which placentas were examined in detail at birth.
2. Toronto Twin Register David Hewitt, PhD Ms. Jean Milner Dept. of Preventive Medicine and Biostatistics University of Toronto Toronto, Canada M5S 1A1 Ph: (416) 978-2058	To provide support for a broad spectrum of twin studies.	Zygosity data and special data from a variety of studies including dermatoglyphics and blood lipids on a volunteer twin panel.	207	An indexed bibliography of twin studies is kept which presently contains about 7,000 items.
3. Winnipeg Women's Center Twin Births Ms. Marion Lewis Dept. of Pediatrics University of Manitoba 735 Notre Dame Ave. Winnipeg, Canada R3E 0L8	To study transfusion syndromes and chimerism as well as provide assistance for twin studies.	Gross placental data and blood typing on twins and parents from a series of twins born from 1963 to 1976.	458	A consecutive series of twins ascertained at birth.
United States				
4. Kaiser-Permanente Twin Registry Gary D. Friedman, MD Dept. of Medical Methods Research Kaiser-Permanente Medical Care Program 3700 Broadway Oakland, CA 94611	Identify and assess environmental and genetic factors in health and disease.	Questionnaire data on a variety of diseases and exposures to potential health hazards are being collected in 1977.	8,000	Register developed since 1975. All ages and races, mostly subscribers to The Kaiser Foundation Health Plan.
5. Rocky Mountain Twin Registry W.J. Kimberling, PhD Dept. of Pediatrics University of Colorado Medical School Denver, CO Ph: (303) 394-8802	A resource for investigators whose research is suited to the twin model.	Family and medical histories on twins from Colorado and Wyoming.	73	

TABLE 2 (Continued)

Register	Purpose of research	Data recorded and source of twins	Total number of twin pairs	Remarks
6. University of Colorado Inst. for Behavioral Genetics Twin Studies Steven G. Vanderberg, PhD and Robert Plomin, PhD Inst. for Behavioral Genetics University of Colorado Boulder, CO 80309 Ph: (303) 492-7362	Studies of behavior in children with emphasis on personality development and logic.	Test data on volunteers from the Denver, Colorado area.	120	Panel just being developed.
7. Connecticut Twin Registry Merton S. Honeyman, PhD Div. of Health Statistics State Dept. of Health 79 Elm Street Hartford, CT 06115 Ph: (203) 566-5975	Twin studies of chronic disease.	Connecticut birth records.	25,000 +	Multiple births in Connecticut have been recorded from July 1, 1897 to present.
8. A Prospective Study: Blood Pressure in Newborn Twins. Henry Gelband, MD, and Robert S. Levine, MD Dept. of Pediatrics University of Miami P.O. Box 520875 Biscayne Annex Miami, FL 33152 Ph: (305) 547-6991	To estimate the genetic component of variance for blood pressure during the first year of life.	Blood pressure, weight, height, and pulse serially for the first year. Dermatoglyphics and placental data including injection studies twins born at The Jackson Memorial–Univ. of Miami Medical Center.	56	Panel just being developed.
9. Ovarian Failure in Monozygotic and Dizygotic Twins Paul G. McDonough, MD Dept. Ob-Gyn Medical College of Georgia Augusta, GA 30902	To understand the etiology of ovarian failure with normal chromosomes.	Georgia and South Carolina.		Twins are being ascertained with pure gonadal dysgenesis.
10. Indiana University Twin Studies Joe C. Christian, PhD, MD Dept. of Medical Genetics Indiana Univ. School of Med. 1100 W. Michigan Indianapolis, IN 46202 Ph: (317) 264-2241	Support for a broad spectrum of twin studies with special emphasis on quantitative studies of coronary heart disease risk factors.	Blood pressure, cholesterol, height, weight, dermatoglyphics, and some placental data on Indiana twins.	906	

11.	Louisville Twin Study Ronald S. Wilson, PhD Univ. of Louisville School of Medicine P.O. Box 1055 Louisville, KY 40201 Ph: (502) 588-5137	Longitudinal study of mental development, and assessment of infant temperament.	Sequential test data, family interviews, behavioral ratings, anthropometric, etc. from 3 months to 9 years of age from Louisville, Kentucky twins.	467	350 sibs from the twin families also tested.
12.	Tulane University Twin Studies H.W. Kloepfer, PhD Dept. of Anatomy Tulane University New Orleans, LA 70112 Ph: (504) 585-5132	Genetic studies of dermatoglyphics.	Dermatoglyphics on twins ascertained from Europe, Canada, U.S.A. and Australia.	800	Data collected in collaboration with Twin Clubs and Mothers of Twins Clubs.
13.	Twin Registry for Eye Examination J.T. Schwartz, MD, MPH Div. of Hospitals and Clinics, USPHS Room 1177 6525 Belcrest Rd. W. Hyattsville, MD 20708 Ph: (301) 436-6215	Heritability and co-twin control studies of eye development and collaborative studies of other organ systems.	Medical history, physical exams, and dermatoglyphics on volunteer twins, most under age 20.	650	
14.	NINCDS Collaborative Perinatal Project Twin Cohort Ntinos C. Myrianthopoulos, PhD Developmental Neurology Branch Natl. Inst. Health Bethesda, MD 20014 Ph: (301) 496-5821	Study of congenital malformations in twins, relationship to placental type, and intellectual development to age 7 years.	Family and socioeconomic history, pregnancy history, placentation, physical and mental parameters of the twins from 55,000 pregnancies.	615	Placental examinations done both by gross and microscopic examinations.
15.	National Academy of Sciences, Natl. Research Council Twin Registry Zdnek Hrubec, PhD Medical Follow-up Agency Natl. Acad. Sci. 2101 Constitution Ave., NW Washington, DC 20418	Provide a resource for a broad program of medical, genetic, epidemiologic, and behavioral studies on adult male twins.	Questionnaire data, military and VA records, fingerprints, and data from special studies. Twins all veterans of U.S. armed forces.	15,924	This panel is available to outside investigators for collaborative studies.

TABLE 2 (Continued)

	Register	Purpose of research	Data recorded and source of twins	Total number of twin pairs	Remarks
16.	Diabetes and Twins J. Stuart Soeldner, MD 1 Joslin Place Boston, MA 02215 Ph: (617) 732-2530	To describe and delineate the genetic component of diabetes mellitus.	Medical records of Joslin Clinic.	250	Extensive genetic markers to be done. Evaluation of carbohydrate tolerance and hormonal responses in unaffected MZ twins.
17.	Research in Psychologic and Psychiatric Genetics I.I. Gottesman, PhD Behavioral Genetics Center Elliot Hall Univ. of Minnesota Minneapolis, MN 55455 Ph: (612) 373-3422	Studies of psychologic and psychiatric genetics.	Psychologic data and psychiatric histories on twins from established registers in U.S., England, and Denmark.		A broad spectrum of collaborative studies with several established twin registers.
18.	Hemoglobinopathies in Twins Michael K. McCormack, MD Dept. of Pediatrics Rutgers Medical School Piscataway, NJ 08854 Ph: (201) 564-4287	Study growth and development in children with hemoglobinopathies.	Medical record data, family data, and psychologic testing on twins referred to Rutgers Medical School and Philadelphia Children's Hospital.		A newly established program.
19.	Obesity in Twins Fredda Ginsberg-Fellner, MD Dept. of Pediatrics Mount Sinai School of Medicine New York, NY 10029	Study of the prevalence and causes of obesity in twins.	Birth history, family history, placental data on twins referred from Mothers of Twins Clubs.	500	
20.	State University of New York Twin Study Larry Green, DDS, PhD Dept. of Orthodontics School of Dentistry State Univ. of New York at Buffalo Buffalo, NY 14214 Ph: (716) 831-2845	A study of craniofacial development.	Dental casts, cephalometric, panorex, and carpal radiographs along with anthropometric data on volunteer twins aged 6 to 14.	200	Not actively recruiting twins since 1970.
21.	Medical College of Virginia Human Twin Panel Walter E. Nance, MD, PhD Dept. of Human Genetics Medical College of Virginia Richmond, VA 23298 Ph: (804) 770-4646	Development of a population-based twin panel for a broad spectrum of twin studies.	Vital statistics and questionnaire data on twins from Virginia and Norway.	30,000 +	One subset of this panel is a consecutive series of newborn twins with placental data.

REFERENCES

1. MacGillivray I, Nylander PPS, Corney G: "Human Multiple Reproduction." Philadelphia: WB Saunders, 1975.
2. Myrianthopoulos NC: In Bergsma D (ed): "Congenital Malformations in Twins: Epidemiologic Survey." Miami: Symposia Specialists for The National Foundation – March of Dimes BDOAS XI(8), 1975.
3. Emery AEH, Miller JR (eds): "Registers for the Detection and Prevention of Genetic Disease." New York: Stratton Intercontinental Medical Book Corp., 1976.
4. Sokal RR, Rohlf FJ: "Biometry." San Francisco: WH Freeman, 1969.
5. Christian JC, Kang KW, Norton JA Jr: Choice of an estimate of genetic variance from twin data. Am J Hum Genet 26:154–161, 1974.
6. Christian JC, Norton JA Jr: A proposed test of the difference between the means of monozygotic and dizygotic twins. Acta Genet Med Gemellol (Roma) 26:49–54, 1977.
7. Havlik R, Garrison R, Fabsitz R, Feinleib M: Genetic variability of clinical chemical values. Clin Chem 23:659–662, 1977.
8. Christian JC, Feinleib M, Norton JA Jr, Kang KW: Quantitative genetic analysis of twin data. Paper presented at the Joint Meeting of the Eastern North American Regional Biometrics Society and the American Statistical Society, St. Paul, Minnesota, March 1975.
9. Reed R, Sprague FR, Kang KW, Nance WE, Christian JC: Genetic analysis of dermatoglyphic patterns in twins. Hum Hered 25:263–275, 1975.
10. Holt SB: "The Genetics of Dermal Ridges." Springfield: Charles C Thomas, 1968.
11. Reed T, Uchida IA, Christian JC: Dermatoglyphic variation in monozygotic twins of differing placental types. In "Fifth International Congress of Human Genetics, Mexico City." Excerpta Medica International Congresses Series 397:37, 1976.
12. Bulmer MG: "The Biology of Twinning in Man." Oxford: Clarendon Press, 1970.
13. Strong SJ, Corney G: The placenta in twin pregnancy. Oxford: Pergamon Press, 1967.
14. Byron E, Slavin B: Serum IgG levels in feto-fetal transfusion syndrome. Arch Dis Child 49:908–910, 1974.
15. Corey LA, Kang KW, Christian JC, Norton JA Jr, Harris RE, Nance WE: Effects of chorion type on variation in cord blood cholesterol of monozygotic twins. Am J Hum Genet 28:433–441, 1976.
16. Corey LA, Kang KW, Christian JC, Nance WE: Birthweight in MZ and DZ twins of known placental type. In "Fifth International Congress of Human Genetics, Mexico City." Excerpta Media International Congresses Series 397:178, 1976.
17. Melnick M, Myrianthopoulos NC, Christian JC: Effects of chorion type on variation in IQ of monozygotic twins. Papers presented at the Second International Congress of Twin Studies, Washington, DC, August–September, 1977.
18. Allen G: Models of proband concordance rates for twins in a clinical series. Acta Genet Med Gemellol (Roma) 19:146–149, 1970.
19. Smith C: Concordance in twins: Methods and interpretation. Am J Hum Genet 26:454–466, 1974.
20. Myrianthopoulos NC, Melnick M: Malformations in monozygotic twins: A possible example of environmental influences on the developmental genetic clock. In Dnouye E, Nishimura H (eds): "Gene-Environmental Interaction in Common Diseases." Tokyo: University of Tokyo Press, 1977, pp 206–220.
21. Benirschke K, Kim CK: Multiple pregnancy. N Engl J Med 288:1276–1284, 1329–1336, 1974.

22. Smith DW, Bartlett C, Harrah LM: Monozygotic twinning and the Duhamel anomalad (imperforate anus to sirenomelia): A nonrandom association between two aberrations in morphogenesis. In Bergsma D, Schimke RD (eds): "Cytogenetics, Environment and Malformation Syndromes." New York: Alan R Liss for the National Foundation–March of Dimes, BD:OAS XII(5):53–63, 1976.
23. Nance WE: Anencephaly and spina bifida: An etiologic hypothesis. In Bergsma D (ed): Part VI. "The Nervous System." Baltimore: Williams & Wilkins for The National Foundation–March of Dimes, BD:OAS VII(1):97, 1971.
24. Giroud A: Role possible en cytoplasme au cours de la morphogenese, notamment dans le cas de la gemellite. Acta Genet Med Gemellol (Roma) 24:251–259, 1975.
25. Opitz JM, Summitt RL, Smith DW: The BBB syndrome. Familial telecanthus with associated congenital anomalies. In Bergsma D (ed): Part II. "Malformation Syndromes." New York: The National Foundation–March of Dimes, BD:OAS V(2):86–94, 1969.
26. Summitt RL, Wilroy RS Jr: Further studies of the telecanthus-hypospadias syndrome. Pediatr Res 8 (Program and Abstracts) 422/168, 1974.
27. Ross RB, Coupes TB: Craniofacial morphology in six pairs of monozygotic twins discordant for cleft lip and palate. J Can Dent Assoc 31:149–157, 1965.
28. Van Dyke DL, Palmer CG, Nance WE, Yu PL: Chromosome polymorphism and twin zygosity. Am J Hum Genet (In press).
29. World Health Organization: The use of twins in epidemiological studies: Report of the WHO meeting of investigators in twin studies. Acta Genet Med Gemellol (Roma) 15: 109–128, 1966.
30. World Health Organization: "WHO International Survey of Twin Registers and Studies." Geneva: WHO, 1966.
31. Lynch WT: "International Directory of Genetic Services." 5th Ed. Bergsma D, Lynch HT (eds): White Plains, New York: The National Foundation–March of Dimes, 1977.
32. International Society for Twin Studies. P Parisi Sec Gen; Mendel Institute Piazza Galeno 5, 00161 Rome, Italy.
33. Myrianthopoulos NC: An epidemiologic survey of twins in a large prospectively studied population. Am J Hum Genet 22:611, 1970.

Conjoined Twins: Nosology and Congenital Malformations*

Kurt Benirschke, MD, William W. Temple, MD, and Colin M. Bloor, MD

INTRODUCTION

Twinning occurs frequently in human reproduction. The understanding of this phenomenon has greatly added to our knowledge of early embryology and the development of some forms of congenital anomalies. In particular, the phenomenon of conjoined twinning has been of interest to physicians and especially to gemellologists who have derived insight into early embryonic developmental forces [1, 2].

The frequency of human twinning varies from approximately 1 in 30 to 1 in 150 pregnancies and is dependent upon hereditary and environmental factors [3]. It is well understood now that at least two classes of twins exist, fraternal (dizygotic) and identical (monozygotic) twins, a third, intermediate class being doubtful [4]. While environmental and hereditary factors suggest that great variations exist in the fraternal twinning frequency, it is generally accepted that monozygotic (MZ) twinning is a relatively constant phenomenon at 3.5/1,000 pregnancies. Recently, it has been suggested that it too has a hereditary component [5], but more data are needed to affirm this relationship.

The existence of monozygotic twinning in litter-bearing animals and plants can occasionally be verified when appropriate phenotypic markers are found to be identical. Often, however, this is difficult. The existence of conjoined twins has then been suggested to "prove" such occurrences, since this form of twinning is generally held to be a form of incomplete fission of single embryos [2]. Newman gives the previous hypothesis of incomplete fusion of two embryos as

*This work was supported by USPHS Training Grant HL07104.

Birth Defects: Original Series, Volume XIV, Number 6A, pages 179–192

a possible alternative for the development of conjoined twins, a view that was reiterated by Aird [6]. These views and other aspects of the conjoined twinning process will be reviewed briefly.

CONJOINED TWINNING

Distribution

Conjoined twins are found among a wide variety of living species. A number of conjoined plants have been observed and a recent study by Ahmad et al [7] gives the incidence of twinning in soybeans. Of 36,000 seeds germinated, 168 resulted in twins (1 triplet) (0.4/1,000). Of these twins, 38 (0.11%) were completely separated but 130 (0.36%) were partially fused. Thoraco-omphalopagi are reported in a turtle [8], in the rat [9, 10], in a dolphin [11], and in a rabbit [12]. In snakes, double-headed "monsters" have been described repeatedly [13, 14], and Tuli and Singe [15] have reported this anomaly in the chicken. We have recently dissected a diprosopus cat, offspring with three other normal kittens. The anomaly has been seen in pigs [16], the mouse [17], a calf [18], and many other species aside from man. In human reproduction, conjoined twins occur with estimated frequencies varying between 1:33,000 and 1:165,000 births, but much higher incidences have been suggested. Most recently, Bhettay et al [19] have been concerned about an "epidemic of conjoined twins in Southern Africa" as possibly being the result of environmental factors. Others have drawn attention to the unreliability of these figures [20]. A peculiar finding has been that 70% of human conjoined twins are females, and thoracopagus twins (73.4%) are much more common than pygopagus (18.8%), ischiopagus (5.9%), or craniopagus (1.7%) conjoined twins [21].

Etiology

The cause of MZ twinning is unknown and that of conjoined twinning is equally obscure. That these twins are products of incomplete fusion of fraternal twins as earlier surmised must now be dismissed as a possibility. When separate genitalia have been present, these were always of like sex; in the few cytogenetic studies so far undertaken, the chromosomes have always been normal and of like sex [22]; when conjoined twins complicate triplet or quadruplet pregnancy, the former are isosexual, the triplet etc may have different sex [21]; early partially separate twins have been observed in occasional embryologic studies. Finally, conjoined bird twins arise in small eggs, while double-yolked eggs, with their potential for fraternal twins, are large. The single support for the fusion hypothesis comes from a brief note by McFeely [23] on "a Holstein cow with two parasitic limbs attached at the level of the thoracic vertebrae and a characteristic freemartin conformation and genitalia (which) was found to be an XX/XY chimera on leukocyte culture." It has since been learned that early blastocyst fusion can readily be achieved experimentally in rodents and that "whole body chimerae," presumably originating in a similar manner, occur infrequently in a variety of species [24]. This mechanism, however, must be discounted as an etiology of most conjoined twins.

Incomplete splitting of a single embryo is thus the accepted current theory and a few environmental teratogens have been alluded to by Newman [2]. In experimentation with *Tritus,* Spemann found that ligation of fertilized dividing eggs yielded conjoined twins. The application of combined heat and hypoxia at about the time of gastrulation has produced conjoined twins in zebra fish [25]. Conjoined twinning has also been observed in golden hamsters following the treatment of the mothers with different teratologic compounds, which include vitamin A, dimethylsulfoxide, etc [26]. Conjoined twinning has also been experimentally produced in the salmon by crowding [27]. Whatever the agent, a common denominator in all is that the forces used to experimentally produce these abnormalities markedly alter the microclimate around the fertilized ovum. The occurrence of rather large numbers of swine with incomplete twinning prompted a statistical analysis of possible factors by Selby and his collaborators [16]. The results of this study identified no major environmental or genetic factors associated with conjoined twinning in the Missouri swine. Four posteriorly duplicated newborn rabbits were noted in 252 births of the Y-strain at the Jackson Laboratories by Chi and Craig [28]. This frequency was felt to be strong evidence for genetic transmission. On the other hand, there was no twinning in the family or the offspring of Eng and Chang, the most illustrious of all conjoined twins [29]. Hereditary influences upon this process are only weakly supported at present.

Pathogenesis

Since the etiology of conjoined twinning is unknown and teratogens induce the anomaly only infrequently, the morphogenesis of these interesting duplications is poorly understood although frequently discussed. The interested reader must consult the volumes by Newman [1, 2] in order to appreciate the extensive deductive thoughts of classic embryologists. Summing up his experiences, Newman concluded that duplicities arose because of a delay in the congress of symmetric halves during embryonic development.

We have suggested elsewhere that the MZ twinning process is a continuum, spanning the first two weeks of embryonic development [30]. In simple terms, this concept states that a "twinning impetus" affects embryonic development at random during development but that it eventuates in twins only during the first two weeks, the "teratogenic termination period" for twins according to

Schwalbe's concept. Because the embryo has axiated and developed longitudinally sufficiently at the end of this period, it is impossible to split it any longer; instead, the same impetus may result in a variety of anomalies thereafter. According to this concept, any teratogen may be effective in causing twinning and corroboration for this effect is found in the evidence from environmental teratologic experiments cited above. The concept would accept the finding that the MZ twinning frequency is fairly uniformly distributed throughout all races and it accords with the placental findings of twins (Fig. 1). It is suggested that during placentation the impetus may achieve twinning of solid embryonic structures but, once a cavity has formed, it cannot be duplicated by the impetus. Thus, the period for dichorionic twinning extends only over the first two days of development, etc. Studies on large twin placental material show that perhaps 70% of MZ twins have a diamnionic, monochorionic placenta, nearly 30% a dichorionic placenta, and very few are monoamnionic, monochorionic. It is therefore suggested that, as development proceeds, the ability to twin becomes more difficult for an embryo. The finding of a monoamnionic relationship in virtually all conjoined twins and their usually single umbilical cord place their morphogenesis into the terminal period of the twinning schedule, around days 13–15 at a time when the primitive streak and axiation commence. Moreover, considering that

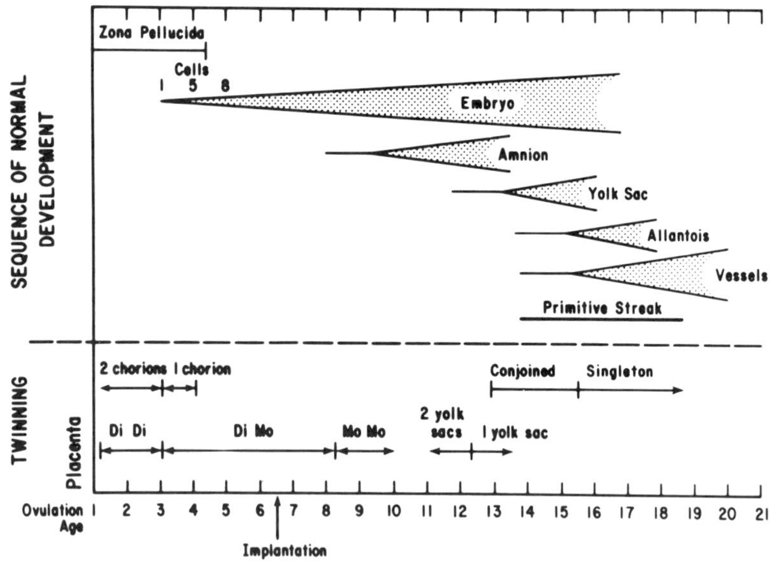

Fig. 1. Schematic representation of early embryonic events to place the origin of twinning. Above are represented the incipient events of differentiation of different embryonic and placental structures; below are the placental membranous relationships assuming that once a cavity is formed, it can no longer be split. As will be seen, because of common amnion and yolk sac, conjoined twins are thought to arise between days 13 and 15. Thereafter the embryo has formed sufficiently that twinning becomes impossible.

somite development begins centrally and spreads caudally and cephalically, the end portions may be able to duplicate later than central portions and thus explain the frequency of anterior and posterior duplications and the excess of thoracopagi.

This (oversimplified) concept could encompass an explanation for the diversification of conjoined twins. Thus, one could construct a developmental table from minimally fused twins to thoracopagi, to those with three legs [31], with two legs [22], and eventually to the diprosopi with only partially split faces, assuming that splitting would become ever more difficult the later the impetus took place. It would accord with ever increasing frequencies of severe congenital anomalies in this hypothetic series. The problem with such a hypothesis is that it does not accord with observations from other species. Thus, among the 67 conjoined pigs studied by Selby et al [16], 35 were syncephali, and only 8 were thoracopagi. Thus, comparative studies of embryologic events in different species may be of great value and, above all, it would be desirable to have an experimental species with predictable frequency of this event. It is possible that the difference in the timing of embryonic implantation into the uterus and different developmental time tables explain the observed differences. Thus, implantation in man occurs around day 6–7, in the pig on day 18; of course, placental development is very different. An interesting unresolved question is why the process of conjoined twinning has not been described or perhaps does not occur in the two species of armadillo with their invariable polyembryony.

Mode of Death

One of the many tales that exist in the twin literature but that pertain particularly to the conjoined twins is that when one of such twins dies, the other is soon to follow. Thus, when Chang died, Eng had premonitions of his impending death although he was perfectly well. Within two hours he died, following a period of anxiety, choking sensation, agonizing leg pains, and profuse diaphoresis [29]. At autopsy no pathologic findings were made in Eng, who was thought to have died from "fright." Aside from some fibromuscular bands, these twins were found to be joined by some liver tissue. The senior author had the opportunity of examining a pair of dicephalus, tetrabrachic twin girls at age 13 in Salvador, Brazil. One twin was nearly laterally attached and suffered from frequent congestive heart failure, the "autosite" being reasonably normal. The normal twin constantly feared demise of the attached twin because it would presumably lead to her own death. This eventually proved to be true. We have previously suggested in monoamnionic twins that placental anastomoses may allow transfer of thromboplastin from a dead twin to initiate disseminated intravascular coagulation in the other [32], a concept supported by other studies [33]. The same may indeed be the cause of death in the second of conjoined twins to die and this possibility should be borne in mind for study and in evaluating the advisability of immediate separation in otherwise appropriate circumstances. In retrospect it is apparent that Eng would have survived had these measures been taken.

Congenital Abnormalities

Congenital anomalies occur more frequently in twins than in singletons, and discordance of anomalies in MZ twins is common, even when a familial or hereditary background for their genesis exists. The subject is complex and has been reviewed on numerous occasions [3] . Discordance of anomalies often affects conjoined twins. Thus, the Brazilian twins suffered tetralogy of Fallot in the "parasite" (A.C. de Queiroz, Bahia; personal communication); anencephaly of one was present in the dicephalus of the patient of Hamon and Dinno [22] ; discordance for cleft lip was described in a thoracopagus by Kim et al [34] ; and numerous other lesions are summarized in a previous monograph by The National Foundation [35] . Perhaps the commonest anomalies exist in the cardiovascular system, and they have attracted the most attention. Despite their frequency and frequent bilaterality, they are never exactly the same in the two twins. The extensive literature has been ably reviewed by de Leon [36] , who describes male thoraco-omphalopagi (with a triplet), a single pericardium and two hearts (one with atrial septal defect, the other with cor biloculare), and a host of other anomalies; de Leon also reviews the frequency (73%) of mirror imagery in conjoined twins, a topic that was of great concern to Newman [37] . The following case reports are of recently observed thoracopagi at this institution. Both had complex cardiac anomalies and died shortly following birth.

CASE REPORTS

Case 1

A one-hour-old set of female monoamnionic thoracopagus twins were delivered by a white, 23-year-old, gravida 1, para 0, woman. The mother was blood group B positive and had a negative serology. The expected date of delivery differed from the premature delivery by 22 days. The diagnosis of twins had been made prior to delivery by fetal heart tones, x-ray examination, and ultrasound study. Forceps were used to deliver twin A, but were not necessary for the delivery of twin B. Twin A initially breathed and had an Apgar rating of 3 at one minute. Twin B had no respiration and had an Apgar score of 0 at one minute. Both twins were intubated. Twin A had an initial heart rate of 40, while there was none in B. Resuscitation efforts were unsuccessful. The combined weight was 4, 350 gm, the placenta weighed 490 gm.

At autopsy the infants were estimated to be at approximately 37 weeks gestation. Both twins were joined from the midsternum to below the umbilicus. There was an inferior omphalocele with a single umbilical cord containing three arteries and one vein. Of these vessels, twin A received one umbilical artery and no umbilical vein, while twin B had two umbilical arteries and one umbilical vein.

Examination of the thoracic cavity showed a common sternum, but normal ribs were present in both twins. Two tracheae, four lungs, and a common pericardial sac were present. Two great vessels extended from each side of the common pericardial sac considered to be the aorta and a pulmonary artery of each twin. After opening the pericardial sac, a common heart was noted (Fig. 2).

Examination of the heart in detail showed that the aorta, arising from the right-sided heart of twin A, was hypoplastic and approximately one-third the size of the pulmonary artery. A right superior vena cava entered the atrium. The azygous vein was present on the right side. A common inferior vena cava entered into the right-sided atrium and the pulmonary vein entered the right superior vena cava above its entrance to the atrium. A normal tricuspid valve was present in the ventricle. There was a double outlet from this right ventricle with a large pulmonary artery arising from the anteriorly located conus region. The pulmonic valve was normal. Beneath the cristae was a small orifice that led into the hypoplastic aorta. There was a large patent ductus arteriosus between the pulmonary artery and aorta of twin A (Figs. 3–5).

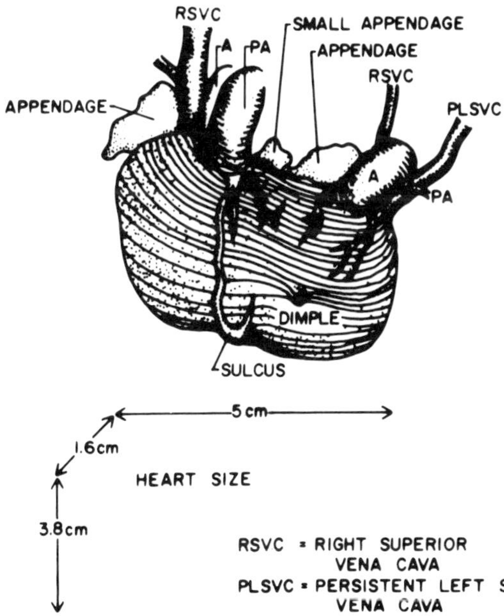

Fig. 2. Common heart and vessels of *Case 1*. A = aorta, PA = pulmonary artery.

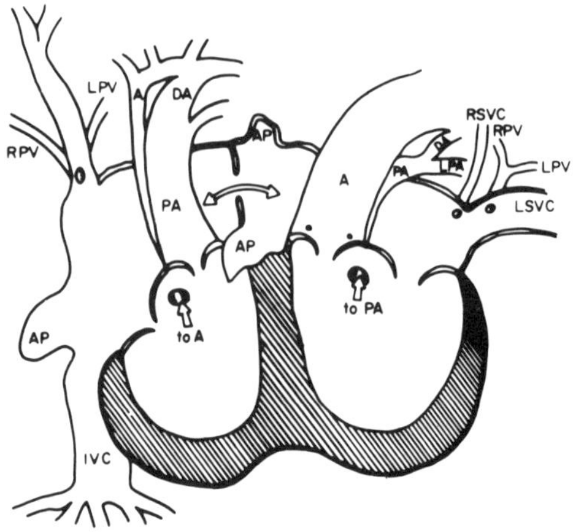

3

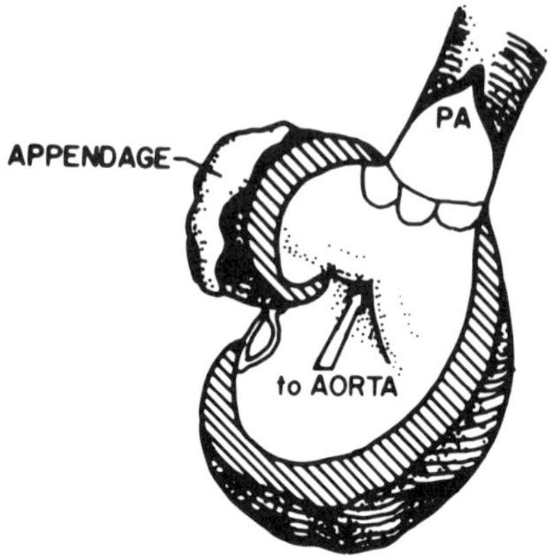

4

Fig. 3. Relationships of chambers and vessels of dissected heart of *Case 1*. IVC = inferior vena cava; AP = atrial appendage; RPV = right pulmonary vein; LPV = left pulmonary vein; A = aorta; PA = pulmonary artery; DA = ductus arteriosus; RSVC = right superior vena cava; LSVC = left superior vena cava.

Fig. 4. View of heart of twin A, *Case 1*. PA = pulmonary artery.

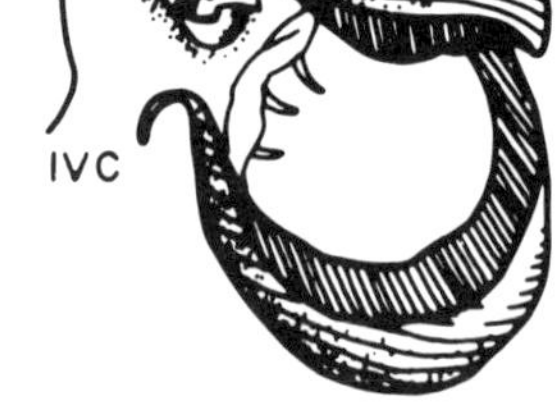

Fig. 5. View of heart of twin A, *Case 1*. IVC = inferior vena cava; RPV = right pulmonary vein; RSVC = right superior vena cava; LPV = left pulmonary vein.

Examination of the heart of twin B showed the aorta and pulmonary artery arising in a transposed fashion, with the aorta located on the right side and slightly anterior to the pulmonary artery. The right and left superior venae cavae entered the left side of the atrium. The right and left pulmonary veins entered the persistent left superior vena cava before it entered the atrium. There was a septal defect or a patent foramen ovale between the two atrial chambers. A normal aortic valve was present. A small opening below the valve led to the pulmonary artery. The pulmonary artery was much smaller than the aorta. A thin thread was present between the junction of the left superior vena cava with the left-sided atrium and resembled a vestigial valve. There was a large patent ductus arteriosus. It is noteworthy that there was no communication between the two ventricular chambers (Figs. 6 and 7).

Both sets of lungs were anatomically normal; however, the lungs of twin B were smaller than those of twin A. Each had a normal thymus. In the peritoneal cavity one diaphragmatic ostium was present for the common inferior vena cava. Each twin had a normal esophagus, stomach, and proximal duodenum. At this point, the duodenum of both infants fused to form a common distal duodenum, which entered a distended loop of common ileum. There was bifurcation of the distal ileum with separate colons (Fig. 8). Each twin had a normal pancreas and spleen; that of twin B was smaller. There was a grossly enlarged common liver. Twin A had a right-sided and twin B had a left-sided gallbladder. Each twin had unremarkable pairs of adrenals, kidneys, ureters, bladder, and reproductive organs. The brains were nearly equally developed.

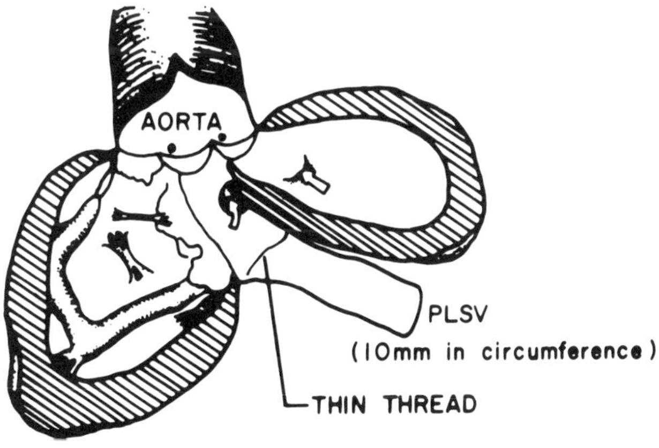

Fig. 6. View of heart of twin B, *Case 1.* PLSV = persistent left superior vena cava.

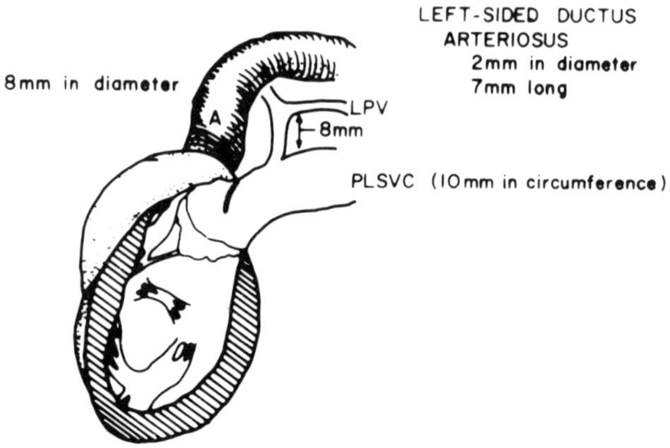

Fig. 7. View of heart of twin B, *Case 1.* LPV = left pulmonary vein; PLSVC = persistent left superior vena cava.

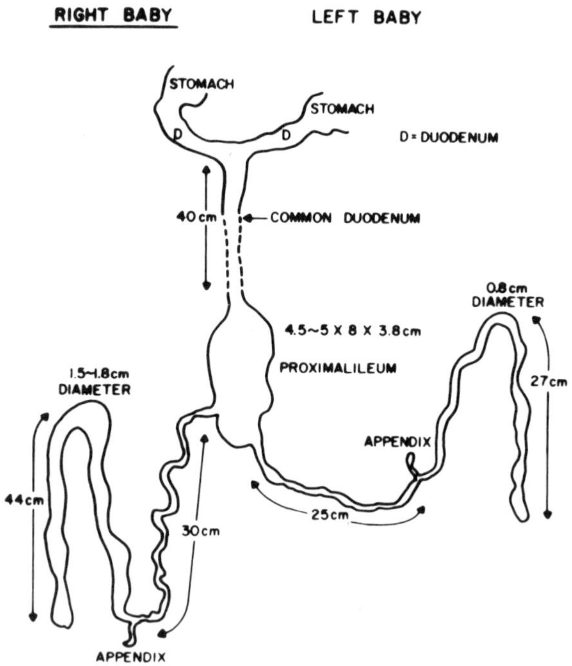

Fig. 8. Relationships of intestinal tracts of *Case 1.*

Case 2

These were a 20-hour-old set of female monoamnionic conjoined twins whose cytogenetic study has previously been reported [34]. At birth twin A had severe respiratory difficulties while twin B was vigorous and had good color. The combined weight was 3,865 gm and there was one umbilical cord with 6 vessels. Only a single set of heart sounds was noted. X-ray study revealed two sets of lungs and a single heart shadow. At cardiac catheterization twin A had a right atrium and right ventricle but there was no evidence of a pulmonary artery, left atrium, or left ventricle. The pulmonary tree in twin A appeared to fill from bronchial vessels. Twin B showed evidence of a right atrium, right ventricle, pulmonary artery, pulmonary vein, left atrium, left ventricle, and aorta. It appeared that there was a common right ventricle or at least a right ventricular defect between twins A and B. It also appeared that twin A's aorta filled from twin B's left ventricle. The twins were intubated. Subsequently, bradycardia and severe respiratory difficulty set in and twin A developed massive subcutaneous emphysema. Respirations became shallow and eventually ceased.

At autopsy there were two complete sets of lungs which appeared to be normal. The heart of twin A had an anatomically normal superior vena cava entering the right atrium, a normal inferior vena cava entering the right atrium, an unremarkable tricuspid valve and right ventricle as well as pulmonary valve and artery. However, there was a large patent ductus arteriosus. The pulmonary veins drained into the left atrium. The left atrium and mitral valve, left ventricle, aortic valve, and aorta were unremarkable. The most unusual feature of the heart of twin A was a small transverse interconnecting vein between B and A. This transverse vein drained into the right atrium. Its origin was not determined (Fig. 9).

Examination of the heart of twin B showed normal superior and inferior venae cavae entering the right atrium. There were tricuspid valvular atresia and a large atrial septal defect. The right ventricle was normally formed, except for a large ventricular septal defect. The pulmonary artery and pulmonary valve were unremarkable except for a large patent ductus arteriosus between aorta and pulmonary artery. The pulmonary veins drained into the left atrium. The mitral valve and left atrium were unremarkable. There was subvalvular stenosis of the aortic valve but the aorta itself was unremarkable.

Each twin had a normal esophagus, except for a small diverticulum in twin B, a normal stomach, and a normal pancreas. The proximal duodenums of both twins were separate; however, the distal portions were fused and there was a common jejunum and proximal ileum. There was bifurcation of this common ileum to form separate distal ileal structures and normal colons. There was a

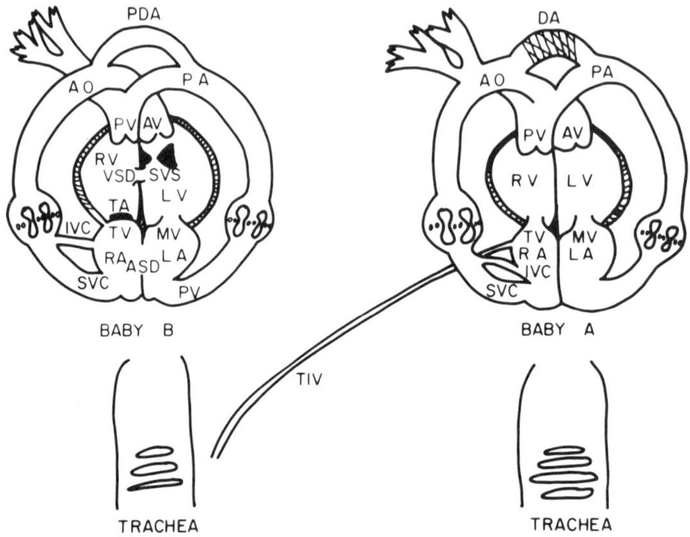

Fig. 9. Cardiac chambers and vessels of twins, *Case 2.* PDA = patent ductus arteriosus; DA = ductus arteriosus; AO = aorta; PA = pulmonary artery; PV = pulmonary valve; AV = aortic valve; RV = right ventricle; LV = left ventricle; VSD = ventricular septal defect; SVS = subvalvular stenosis; TA = tricuspid atresia; TV = tricuspid valve; MV = mitral valve; RA = right atrium; LA = left atrium; IVC = inferior vena cava; SVC = superior vena cava; PV = pulmonary vein; ASD = atrial septal defect; TIV = transverse interconnecting vein.

large fused liver. Injection of the hepatic system showed that there were connecting portal systems. There were no other gross anatomic abnormalities.

FINAL COMMENT

As is so commonly the case, the cardiac anomalies in both these sets of twins were discordant and complex. In reviewing a number of well-described thoracopagus cardiac anomalies, they all differ in some respects from one another, further suggesting that conjoined twins form at different embryologic times. Gilbert et al [38] reviewed relevant thoughts and suggested that these anomalies can best be explained by incomplete fission of the yolk sac [40]. The time table (Fig. 1) supports this view, as does the timing of appearance of the cardiac tube (± 18 d). The proximity of these structures (endoderm, pericardial celom) would lead to various degrees of fusion and separation. It remains to be elucidated what the teratologic force is that engenders the fission in the first place.

REFERENCES

1. Newman HH: "The Biology of Twins." Chicago: University of Chicago Press, 1917.
2. Newman HH: "The Physiology of Twinning." Chicago: University of Chicago Press, 1923.
3. Benirschke K, Kim CK: Multiple pregnancy. N Engl J Med 288:1276–1284, 1329–1336, 1973.
4. Bulmer MG: "The Biology of Twinning in Man." Oxford: Clarendon Press, 1970.
5. Shapiro LR, Zemek L, Shulman MJ: Genetic etiology for monozygotic twinning. This volume.
6. Aird I: Conjoined twins – further observations. Br Med J 1:1313, 1959.
7. Ahmad QN, Britten EJ, Byth DE: Haploid soybeans, a rare occurrence in twin seedlings. J Hered 68:67, 1977.
8. Zabunewicz S, McCready JD: A case of "Siamese" twins in the turtle (Pseudemys scripta elegans). Texas J Sci 19:232–233, 1967.
9. Levinsky HV: A case of conjoined twins in the Sprague-Dawley rat. Lab Anim Sci 23: 903–904, 1973.
10. Cockrell BY: A case of monster twinning (thoracopagus) in the Sprague-Dawley rat (Spartan strain). Lab Anim Sci 22:102–103, 1972.
11. Kawamura A, Kashita K: A rare double monster of dolphin, Stennela caeruleoalba. Sci Rep Whales Res Inst (Tokyo), 23:139–140, 1971.
12. Cock AG: A case of incomplete twinning in a rabbit. J Genet 50:59–60, 1970.
13. Shaw CE: Double troubles again. Zoonooz (San Diego) 41:4–6, 1968.
14. Shaw CE: A two-headed tale. Zoonooz (San Diego) 44:4–7, 1971.
15. Tuli SM, Singe S: Partial anterior duplication (anadidymous) of chick. Congen Anom (Tokyo) 11:15–17, 1971.
16. Selby LA, Khalili A, Stewart RW, Edmonds LD, Marienfeld CJ: Pathology and epidemiology of conjoined twinning in swine. Teratology 8:1–10, 1973.
17. Bateman AJ: Dichorial one-egg twin in the mouse. Nature 187:339–340, 1960.
18. Jenkins TW: Diprosopus and partial cephalic malformations in a calf. Anat Rec 160: 161–170, 1968.
19. Bhettay E, Nelson MM, Beighton P: Epidemic of conjoined twins in Southern Africa. Lancet 2:741–743, 1975.
20. Hanson JW: Incidence of conjoined twinning. Lancet 2:1257, 1975.
21. Rudolph AJ, Michaels JP, Nichols BL: Obstetric management of conjoined twins. In Bergsma D (ed): "Conjoined Twins." New York: The National Foundation–March of Dimes, BD:OAS III (1): 28, 1967.
22. Hamon A, Dinno N: Dicephalus dipus tribrachius conjoined twin in a female infant. This volume.
    Annual Review of Birth Defects (In press).
23. McFeely RM: Aneuploidy, polyploidy and structural rearrangement of chromosomes in mammals other than man. In Benirschke K (ed): "Comparative Mammalian Cytogenetics." New York: Springer-Verlag, 1969, pp 434–444.
24. Benirschke K: Spontaneous chimerism in mammals. A critical review. Curr Top Pathol 51:1–61, 1970.
25. Ingalls TH, Philbrook FR, Majima A: Conjoined twins in zebra fish. Arch Environ Health 19:344–352, 1969.
26. Ferm VH: Conjoined twinning in mammalian teratology. Arch Environ Health 19:353–357, 1969.

27. Stockard CR: Developmental rate and structural expression: An experimental study of twins, "double monsters" and single deformities, etc. Am J Anat 28:155–277, 1921.
28. Chi CK, Craig DD: Conjoined twinning in rabbits. Teratology 4:433–444, 1971.
29. Guttmacher AF: Biographical notes on some famous conjoined twins. In "Conjoined Twins." op cit, pp10–17.
30. Benirschke K, Driscoll SG: "The Pathology of the Human Placenta." New York: Springer-Verlag, 1967.
31. Lichten EM, Teteris NJ: Thoracopagus tripus: An unusual form of conjoined twins. Am J Obstet Gynecol 126:735–737, 1976.
32. Benirschke K: Twin placenta in perinatal mortality. N Y State J Med 61:1499–1508, 1961.
33. Moore CM, McAdams AJ, Sutherland J: Intrauterine disseminated intravascular coagulation: A syndrome of multiple pregnancy with a dead twin fetus. J Pediatr 74:523–528, 1969.
34. Kim CK, Barr RJ, Benirschke K: Cytogenetic studies of conjoined twins. A case report. Obstet Gynecol 38:877–881, 1971.
35. Bergsma D (ed): "Conjoined Twins." op cit, pp 1–147.
36. de Leon F: Siamesische Zwillinge mit differenten Herzmissbildungen. Virchows Arch (Pathol Anat) 362:51–57, 1974.
37. Newman HH: Differences between conjoined twins. In relation to a general theory of twinning. J Hered 22:201–215, 1931.
38. Gilbert EF, Suzuki H, Kimmel DL, Klingberg WG, Lancaster JR: A case of thoracopagus: Conjoined twins. Teratology 6:197–200, 1972.
39. Zimmerman AA: Embryologic and anatomic considerations of conjoined twins. In "Conjoined Twins." op cit, pp 18–27.

A New Tool in Birth Defects Research: The MZ Half-Sib Model and Its Extension to Grandchildren of Identical Twins*

Linda A. Corey, PhD, Walter E. Nance, MD, PhD, and Kare Berg, MD

Numerous studies have documented the importance of both genetic and environmental factors in the etiology of birth defects. Secular and geographic variation in incidence of specific malformations [1] as well as the recognized influence of socioeconomic factors [2] and specific agents such as radiation, drugs, and viral infection during pregnancy clearly emphasize the importance of environmental causes of birth defects. On the other hand, the evidence for a significant familial aggregation of affected individuals with congenital heart disease [3], chromosomal aneuploidy [4], midline neurologic defects [5], clubfoot [6] and many other birth defects provides strong evidence for the etiologic significance of genetic factors. In addition to these two major causes, maternal effects have been implicated in the origin of diabetic embryopathies, the effects on offspring from maternal phenylketonuria (PKU) and certain central nervous system disorders in man [7], and of cleft lip and palate in experimental animals [8]. Maternal effects can be subdivided into those that are attributable to heritable cytoplasmic factors, those that are determined by the nuclear genotype of the mother, and those that are determined by the maternal environment. The last category would include age and parity effects and factors such as maternal diet, smoking habits, or alcohol consumption during pregnancy. Although there

*This is paper #27 of the Department of Human Genetics at the Medical College of Virginia. The Norwegian Twin Register is part of the Central Registry for Inherited Disorders, located at the Institute of Medical Genetics, University of Oslo, and is supported by the Norwegian Research Council for Science and Humanities. It was supported in part by NIH grant #1 PO1 HD 10291-01.

Birth Defects: Original Article Series, Volume XIV, Number 6A, pages 193–200

is strong evidence that genetic, environmental, and maternal effects all play important roles in the etiology of specific birth defects, the designs of previous studies have not permitted an unambiguous assessment of the relative importance of these three types of effects in the determination of the vast majority of common birth defects.

Because many common birth defects appear to have a definite hereditary component, but are not inherited in a simple mendelian fashion and seem to be influenced to some extent by the environment, their etiologies usually have been ascribed to multifactorial inheritance. The multifactorial model assumes that the liability for a given birth defect is continuously distributed and that the actual expression of the defect is determined both by polygenic and environmental factors. The defect is expressed phenotypically if the liability for that malformation exceeds a developmental threshold, either through inheritance or because of environmental exposure, or both. Studies involving a comparison of recurrence risks among different classes of related individuals have provided much of the existing evidence supporting the multifactorial model. Most authors agree, however, that exisiting data and analytic methodologies, including classic twin and family studies, do not permit a clear distinction to be made between this model and the alternative hypothesis that the observed familial aggregation results from single major genes that show reduced penetrance. The distinction is particularly difficult to make when the defect under consideration represents a class of pathologies that are heterogeneous in origin but homogeneous in phenotype. If maternal effects also influence the trait, the problem of assessing the relative importance of genetic and environmental factors may be greatly complicated, and because genetic and maternal effects usually are confounded in conventional family studies, little progress has been made in partitioning human maternal effects into their constituent elements. Thus, the lack of an effective genetic methodology for resolving the genetic, maternal, and environmental components in the etiology of common birth defects has precluded formulation of a clear answer to the question of whether they should be regarded as multifactorial traits or as single-gene defects.

Based on the study of children of identical twins, we have recently developed an analytic methodology that holds great promise for the detection of maternal effects as well as for the resolution of the single major locus versus multifactorial inheritance controversy. Because this half-sib methodology involves data from the children of identical twins rather than from the twins themselves, it circumvents many of the problems usually associated with twin studies but still exploits the unique relationship between monozygotic (MZ) twins. The half-sib method also has many of the advantages of family studies in that several different classes of relatives are present in one family (Fig. 1). In addition to being applicable to the analysis of quantitative traits (Table 1), the half-sib model can be applied to investigate the genetic determination of discontinuous traits. For example,

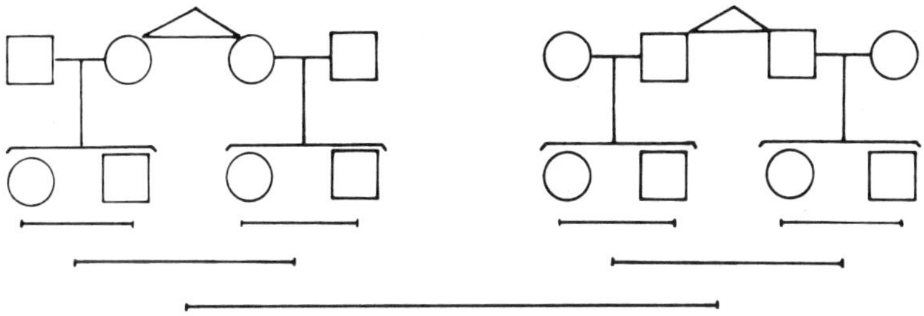

Fig. 1. Structure of MZ half-sib data.

maternal effects can be detected by a comparison of the incidence of birth defects in the children of male versus female identical twins; if the expression of a birth defect is influenced by maternal factors, the incidence of the malformation in the children of a female twin would be higher than that in the children of a male twin.

Through a comparison of the recurrence of specific malformations among children of MZ co-twins (half-sibs) with that observed in the children of the index twin (full-sibs), one can determine if the multifactorial model does, in fact, explain the etiology of the trait in question. If a specific malformation is multifactorial in origin, both parents should, on the average, contribute equally to genetic liability in the children, and one would therefore expect the recurrence in full-sibs to be more than twice as great as that observed among half-sibs. However, if the malformation were to originate from a dominant gene with reduced penetrance, there would be an equal probability that the gene was carried by either the index twin or his or her spouse, and thus the recurrence among children of the co-twin should, on the average, be exactly half that observed among children of the index twin. The model and methodology used in examining identical twins and their families have previously been presented in detail [9].

Although the MZ half-sib model provides a unique and powerful tool in understanding the etiology of common birth defects, it is limited in the extent to which it can partition maternal effects when they are observed. To overcome this limitation, we have extended the model to include the grandchildren of identical twins.

The grandchildren of MZ twins are related to one another in the same way as 1½ cousins (Fig. 2). Just as data on the children of MZ twins can be examined with respect to a quantitative trait like birthweight, so the observed variation in the grandchildren can be partitioned by a nested analysis of variance involving two levels of nesting (Table 2), and the genetic, environmental, and maternal constituents of the resulting variance components can be specified (Table 3). There are 20 distinct types of 1½ cousinships based upon the sexes of the twin grandparents, parents, and grandchildren (Fig. 3).

TABLE 1. Analysis of Variance of Half-Sib Data

Source of variation	Degree of freedom	Mean square	Expected mean square
Among half-sibships	N–1	MSA	$\sigma^2_W + b_2\sigma^2_B + a\sigma^2_A$
Between sibships– within half-sibships	N	MSB	$\sigma^2_W + b_1\sigma^2_B$
Within sibships	$\Sigma(n_i^{1} \; ; n_i^{2}) - 2N$	MSW	σ^2_W
Total	$\Sigma(n_i^{1} + n_i^{2}) - 1$	MST	

$$b_1 = \frac{\Sigma(n_{i1} + n_{i2}) - [\Sigma(n_{i1}^2 + n_{i2}^2)/(n_{i1} + n_{i2})]}{N} \qquad b_2 = \frac{\Sigma(n_{i1}^2 + n_{i2}^2)/(n_{i1} + n_{i2}) - [\Sigma(n_{i1}^2 + n_{i2}^2)/\Sigma(n_{i1} + n_{i2})]}{N-1}$$

$$a = \frac{\Sigma(n_{i1} + n_{i2}) - [\Sigma(n_{i1} + n_{i2})^2/\Sigma(n_{i1} + n_{i2})]}{N-1}$$

TABLE 2. Analysis of Variance for Data From the Grandchildren of Identical Twins*

Source of variation	Degrees of freedom	E(MS)
Among 1½ cousinships	N – 1	$\sigma^2_W + S_3\sigma^2_{BS} + C_2\sigma^2_{BC} + a\sigma^2_A$
Between first cousinships nested within 1½ cousinships	N	$\sigma^2_W + S_2\sigma^2_{BS} + C_1\sigma^2_{BC}$
Between full sibships nested within first cousinships	2N	$\sigma^2_W + S_1\sigma^2_{BS}$
Within full sibships	$\Sigma(n_{ij1} + n_{ij2}) - 4N$	σ^2_W

*Model given assumes a symmetric design with two fertile offspring for each twin but unequal sibship size among the grandchildren. (N = number of 1½ cousinships; n = number of grandchildren in each sibship.)

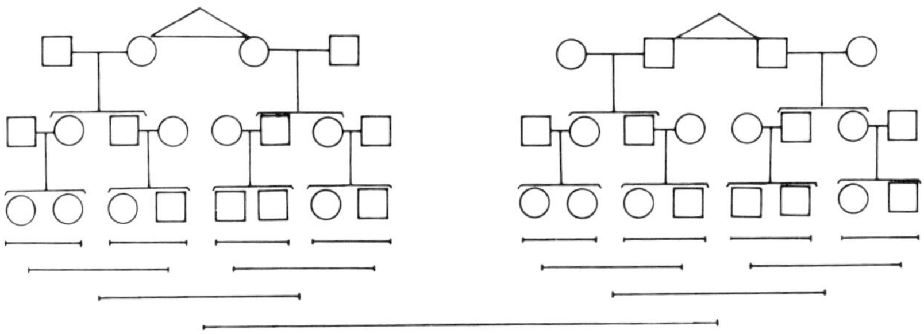

Fig. 2. Structure of data of grandchildren of identical twins.

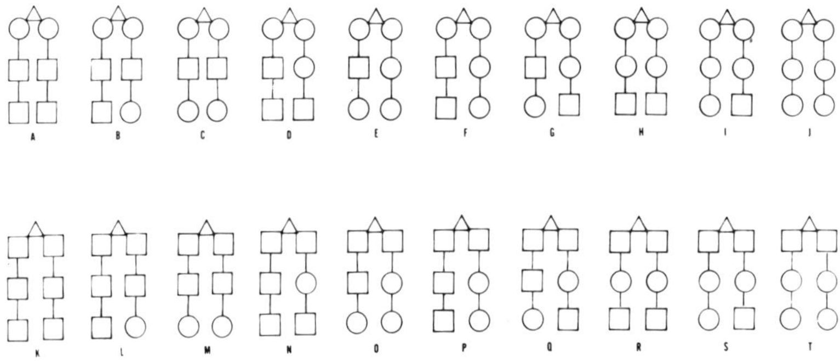

Fig. 3. Twenty distinct 1½ cousins relationships among the grandchildren of MZ twins.

We believe that the present model in conjunction with the previously described MZ twin half-sib relationships provides a powerful and definitive set of equations for the analysis of quantitative inheritance in man. In particular, the equations permit a clear resolution of maternal effects resulting from nuclear, cytoplasmic, and environmental factors, respectively. If it is assumed 1) that the female parent is the sole contributor of the cytoplasmic DNA to the zygote, 2) that the nuclear genotype of the female has no permanent effect on the constitution of cytoplasmic DNA of the germ cells transmitted from generation to generation, and 3) that cytoplasmic traits remain stable and do not segregate when transmitted from one generation to the next, then all the matrilineal grandchildren (1½ cousins) of a female identical twin pair (Fig. 2), for example, should share identical cytoplasms, whereas the patrilineal grandchildren (1½ cousins) of a female identical twin pair would have no cytoplasmic factors in common. Therefore, if the expression of a specific birth defect were influenced by the cytoplasm, one would expect to see a higher incidence of the defect among other matrilineal grandchildren of an index twin than that among the patrilineal grandchildren.

Comparisons of the incidence of birth defects in patrilineal and matrilineal grandchildren of male and female identical twins will permit the detection of both cytoplasmic and maternal influences as well as their formal resolution from X-linked gene effects. Moreover, comparisons of variation in quantitative traits among and within families of the children of identical twins will permit a clearer resolution of the genetic and environmental components of variance than that provided by the half-sib model.

Table 3 gives the genetic, cytoplasmic, maternal, and environmental expectations for four selected nested analyses of variance of grandchildren of identical twins. The between-full-sibship–within-first-cousinship (I-BS) partition for patrilineal grandchildren of male identical twins contains variation resulting from both cytoplasmic and genetically determined maternal effects: in this situation all of the similarities of sibs attributable to maternal effects are determined by women who are genetically unrelated. On the other hand, the variation resulting from cytoplasmic effects in matrilineal grandchildren of male identical twins appears in the between-cousinship–within-1½-cousinship partition of variance (II-BC): in these families there is no variation in cytoplasmic effects within cousins since they arise from women who are full sisters. Finally, in the matrilineal grandchildren of female identical twins, variation resulting from cytoplasmic effects occurs only in the among-1½-cousinship partition of variance (III-A), since, in this case, there should be no variation at all in cytoplasmic effects within the entire kinship. As shown in Table 3, the distribution of genetically determined maternal effects depends upon whether the mothers of the grandchildren are related. A simultaneous solution of these equations will permit the direct estimation of the genetic and cytoplasmic components of the maternal variance as well as the direct genetic (V_A, V_D, etc) and environmental variances. The extended model also removes any biases that might be introduced by the inclusion of the multigenerational comparisons, since the grandchildren's equations provide sufficient information to confine the analysis to individuals who are members of the same generation, thus eliminating the need to include parent–offspring regressions in the analysis.

The models discussed above provide a unique and effective tool for investigating the etiology of common birth defects. Regardless of the complexity of analytical methods, there is a practical limit to the genetic inferences that can be drawn from data from nuclear families such as identical twins reared apart or adoptive children. Eaves has shown that, when a quantitative genetic analysis is confined to relationships in which the parameters to be estimated are largely confounded, an enormous amount of data may be required to detect significant effects [10]. The power of the MZ half-sib model and the extension presented here is that the relationships that exist within these families provide

TABLE 3. Expectations for Nested Analyses of Selected Offspring of Children of Male and Female MZ Twins*

PARTITION	VARIANCE COMPONENT	V_A	V_D	V_{AA}	V_{DD}	V_{AD}	V_{AM}	V_{DM}	V_C	V_{EC}	V_{EF}	V_{ES}	V_{EW}
I. PATRILINEAL GRANDCHILDREN OF MALE IDENTICAL TWINS 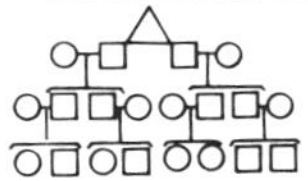													
Among 1½ Cousinships	σ^2_A	1/16	0	1/256	0	0	0	0	0	1	0	0	0
Between First Cousins/ 1½ Cousinships	σ^2_{BC}	1/16	0	3/256	0	0	0	0	0	0	1	0	0
Between Full Sibs/ First Cousinships	σ^2_{BS}	3/8	1/4	15/64	1/16	1/8	1	1	1	0	0	1	0
Within Full Sibships	σ^2_W	1/2	3/4	3/4	15/16	7/8	0	0	0	0	0	0	1
II. MATRILINEAL GRANDCHILDREN OF MALE IDENTICAL TWINS 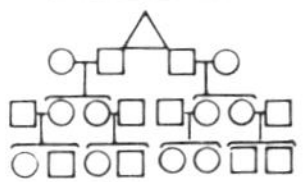													
Among 1½ Cousinships	σ^2_A	1/16	0	1/256	0	0	1/4	0	0	1	0	0	0
Between First Cousins/ 1½ Cousinships	σ^2_{BC}	1/16	0	3/256	0	0	1/4	1/4	1	0	1	0	0
Between Full Sibs/ First Cousinships	σ^2_{BS}	3/8	1/4	15/64	1/16	1/8	1/2	3/4	0	0	0	1	0
Within Full Sibships	σ^2_W	1/2	3/4	3/4	15/16	7/8	0	0	0	0	0	0	1
III. MATRILINEAL GRANDCHILDREN OF FEMALE IDENTICAL TWINS 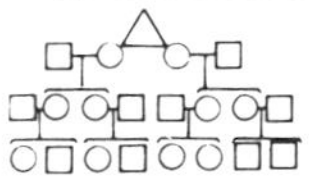													
Among 1½ Cousinships	σ^2_A	1/16	0	1/256	0	0	1/4	0	1	1	0	0	0
Between First Cousins/ 1½ Cousinships	σ^2_{BC}	1/16	0	3/256	0	0	1/4	1/4	0	0	1	0	0
Between Full Sibs/ First Cousinships	σ^2_{BS}	3/8	1/4	15/64	1/16	1/8	1/2	3/4	0	0	0	1	0
Within Full Sibships	σ^2_W	1/2	3/4	3/4	15/16	7/8	0	0	0	0	0	0	1

*V_A = component of additive genetic variance; V_D = component of dominance variance; V_{AA} = component of epistatic interaction between additive effects; V_{DD} = component of epistatic interaction between dominance effects; V_{AD} = component of epistatic interaction between additive and dominance effects; V_{AM} = component of additive maternal effects; V_{DM} = component of dominance maternal effects; V_C = cytoplasmic effects; V_{EC} = effect of environment associated with 1½ cousinships; V_{EF} = effects of environment associated with first cousinships; V_{ES} = effect of environment associated with full sibships; V_{EW} = environmental variance within full sibships.

multiple equations and contrasts in which additive, dominance, maternal, and environmental effects are not confounded.

To apply the new method to the analysis of relatively rare events such as birth defects, a large sample of male and female identical twins will be required. Fortunately, a large twin registry exists in Norway. Systematic collection of the reproductive histories of approximately 8,000 adult MZ twin pairs born in Norway since 1915 and of 12,000 adult offspring of these twins will provide data on approximately 50,000 births in three large data sets. Older twins will yield data on their half-sib offspring as well as grandchildren. Younger twins will yield additional half-sib data that are contemporaneous with the previous set of data on grandchildren, thereby permitting the detection of systematic environmental differences from one generation to the next by comparing the two sets of half-sib data.

The half-sib model and its extension to the grandchildren of identical twins should answer several important questions concerning the etiology and expression of common birth defects and could lead to the identification and resolution of previously unrecognized types of maternal effects that may be of importance in the genesis of certain malformations.

REFERENCES

1. Stevenson AC, Johnson HA, Stewart MIP, Golding DR: Congenital malformations. Bull WHO 34 (Suppl):1, 1966.
2. Janerich DT: Maternal factors in C.N.S. malformations: The cohort approach. In Janerich DT, Skalko RG, Porter IH (eds): "Congenital Defects: New Directions in Research." New York: Academic Press, 1974, p 73.
3. Nora JJ, Meyer TC: Familial nature of congenital heart disease. Pediatrics 37:329, 1966.
4. Alberman E, Elliott M, Creasy M, Dhadial R: Previous reproductive history in mothers presenting with spontaneous abortions. Br J Obstet Gynaecol 82:366, 1975.
5. Williamson EM: Incidence and family aggregation of major congenital malformations of the central nervous system. J Med Genet 2:161, 1965.
6. Palmer RM, Conneally PM, Yu PC: Studies of the inheritance of idiopathic talipes equinovarus. Orthop Clin North Am 5:99, 1974.
7. Fedrick J: Anencephalus: Variation with maternal age, parity, social class and region in England, Scotland and Wales. Ann Hum Genet 34:31, 1970.
8. Fraser FC: Some aspects of maternal effects on congenital malformations. In "Congenital Defects: New Directions in Research." op cit p 17.
9. Nance WE, Corey LA: Genetic models for the analysis of data from the families of identical twins. Genetics 83:811, 1976.
10. Eaves LJ: Computer simulation of sample size and experimental design in human psychogenetics. Psychol Bull 77:144, 1972.

Twin Recurrence and Amniocentesis: Male and MZ Heritability Factors*

Virginia V. Michels, MD and Vincent M. Riccardi, MD

INTRODUCTION

Amniocentesis for genetic indications has become a routine part of obstetric health care for many couples [1]. Yet if twins are unrecognized at the time of amniocentesis the usefulness of analysis of amniotic fluid may be mitigated [2]. The cost of this approach to disease prevention is often $500.00 or more per case, reflecting the utilization of multiple techniques, including ultrasound examination of the uterine contents. Although ultrasonography has many benefits, including placental localization, estimation of gestational age, detection of neural tube defects and recognition of twins [1], it is not applied uniformly [3], at least in part because it is relatively expensive (ie $60.00–$100.00). In order to determine whether family history data regarding twins among genetic relatives to the pregnant couple might indicate when ultrasound should be used, we analyzed information derived from families ascertained on the basis of twin offspring.

Traditionally, the familial recurrence of twins has been considered important only for dizygotic (DZ) twins, and then only when mediated through maternal factors [4]. Our preliminary assessments suggested that monozygotic (MZ) twins and paternal factors may also be important and recently data published by Harvey and co-workers [5] have corroborated this impression.

We demonstrate here that, in at least some families, the presence of multiple MZ or DZ twins among relatives of either parent may forecast the recurrence of

*Dr. Michels is supported by NIGMS training grant GM-00081/03 and Dr. Riccardi is supported in part by the Muscular Dystrophy Association.

Birth Defects: Original Article Series, Volume XIV, Number 6A, pages 201–211

twins among their offspring. In the context of such positive family histories, ultrasound diagnostic techniques should be an integral part of the prenatal diagnostic process.

MATERIALS AND METHODS

The primary study population (Group I) was derived from the active membership of two Milwaukee, Wisconsin lay organizations known as the Milwaukee Mothers of Twins Club and the Organization of Twin-Blessed Mothers. Coordinated by their research chairperson, Ms. G. Giesige, 70 of 200 members responded to a questionnaire inquiring about all known twin pairs in the family, their zygosity, and relationships. When feasible, incomplete preliminary responses were followed up to make the completeness comparable from one family to another. In all instances at least a partial pedigree was constructed to demonstrate the genetic relationship between twin pairs. There was no mechanism to determine any differences between responders and nonresponders. Nor was it determined formally what distinguished members of one of the two organizations from nonmember parents of twins, although awareness of multiple sets of twins in each family was one apparent bias. There were no instances of twins following the use of ovulation-inducing drugs (eg clomiphene). Birth orders, parental ages, and maternal parity were known in only several instances.

Twins were considered to be MZ only if stipulated specifically by the parents; these instances have been designated in Figures 1–6 by diverging lines connected by a horizontal bar (A); all other twins have been designated merely by diverging lines (Λ). Although DZ twinning was considered certain only when the pair was of unlike sex or there were distinct karyotypes (ie one pair discordant for trisomy 21), the phrase "DZ twins" is applied whenever monozygosity is not stipulated.

Two other study populations were derived to serve as controls. Group II comprised a random sampling of 60 families referred for genetic counseling at the Genetics Unit, Milwaukee Children's Hospital, from October 1975 through January 1977. This group indicated how many families have twins if the proband is not a twin and families are not selected for twinning. Group III was obtained from the Birth Defects–Genetic Counseling Clinic, Baylor College of Medicine. The 70 families in this group were ascertained from a sampling of families seen in the clinic during June 1967 through March 1977. The purpose of this group was to assess the clustering of twins in families, without the bias of twin probands ascertained because they are twins but where twins happened to serve as the index case for inclusion in our study. Clinic records were sampled randomly until 70 families, characterized by the presence of one or more twin sets, were identified.

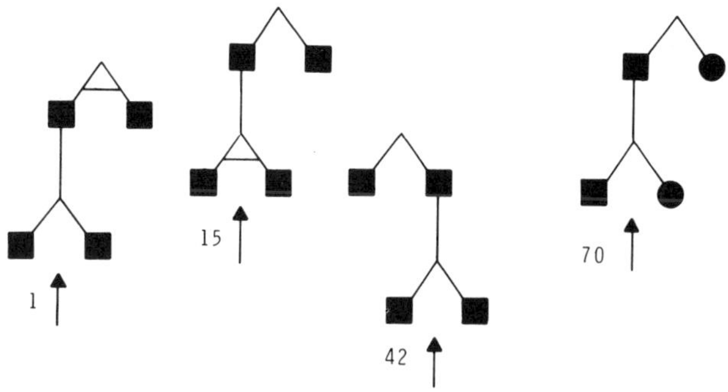

Fig. 1. Representative pedigrees suggesting inheritance factor for twinning transmitted through a male. Note discordance of zygosity in families 1 and 15.

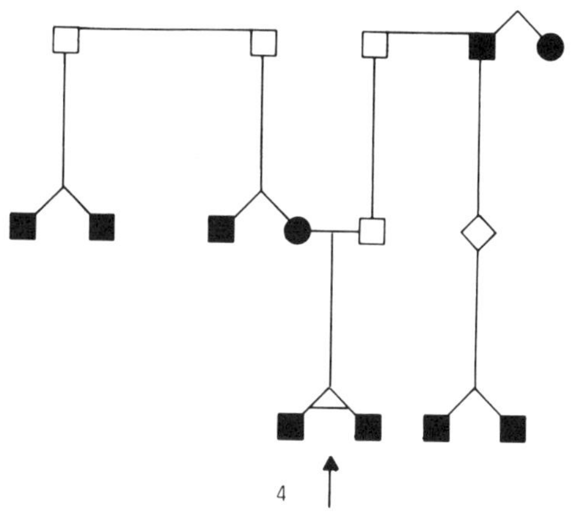

Fig. 2. Representative pedigree suggesting heritability of twinning directly through the paternal side of the family and through male ancestors on the maternal side.

Data from all three groups were compiled in terms of the numbers of families positive for twinning events and the number of twin sets per family. Our main focus was on the presence and magnitude of family clustering although frequency rates for each group of families, and selected subgroups, were derived.

RESULTS

The basic data derived from Group I are indicated in Tables 1–3, and representative pedigrees are depicted in Figures 1–6. Of 70 proband twin sets, 17 were said to be MZ (24%) and 53 were considered to be DZ (76%) (Table 1). Both MZ and DZ twin sets were present in 20 of 52 (34%) families in which there were at least 2 twin sets, and in 14 of 32 (44%) in which there were at least 3 twin sets. In addition to the 16 families containing both monozygotic and dizygotic twins noted in Table 1, there were 4 families in which twins of different zygosity were noted for more distant relatives (eg Fig. 3). Although zygosity was not rigidly established, the data were viewed as being comparable in accuracy to the majority of histories that would be obtained in a counseling session prior to amniocentesis. The presence of both types of twins in a given family is illustrated in Figures 1 through 5.

It was also noted that male intermediaries were present in 31 of the 52 families with positive histories and in 21 of 32 (66%) families with 3 or more twin sets. Of the latter group, there were 8 instances (25%) in which a male was a critical genetic intermediary between related twin sets (Figs. 2–5); in another 13 families (41%) a male intermediary was noted, and his wife also had twin relatives through at least one male (*Family 51,* Fig. 5). In a final instances, in addition to a paternal factor, a non-male-mediated maternal factor was also present. In only 6 of the 32 families (19%) was no paternal influence suggested.

TABLE 1. Proportions (%) of 70 Families of Group I With Related Twins*

Nearest related twin set:		Zygosity of probands		Totals	
Relation	Zygosity	MZ	DZ	No.	%
None	–	3	12	15	21
1°	MZ	0	1	5	7
	DZ	2	2		
2°	MZ	1	1	17	24
	DZ	4	11		
3°	MZ	2	3	14	20
	DZ	1	8		
4°	MZ	0	1	16	23
	DZ	3	12		
Other	–	1	2	3	4
Totals		17	53	70	100

*Nearest related twin set indicates closest twin relatives to proband twin set.

TABLE 2. Excess Numbers of Twin Sets in Group I*

Twin set relatedness	Total no. of families (a)	No. of families with excess (b)	No. excessive twin sets (c)	Average excess: For total subgroup (c/a)	Average excess: For those with excess (c/b)
1°	5	1	3	0.60	3.00
2°	17	12	33	1.94	2.75
3°	14	8	9	0.64	1.13
4°	16	11	29	1.81	2.64
Totals	52	32	74	1.42	2.31

*Excess twin sets are defined as those beyond the proband twin set and closest relative twin set; ie all twins in a family beyond the first two sets.

TABLE 3. Proportions (%) of Families With One or More Twin Sets, and Degree of Relationship to Proband or Index Case*

	None	1°	2°	3°	4°	Other
Group I	21	7	24	20	23	4
Group II	75	7	5	5	8	0
Group III	76	10	9	6	0	0

*Group I is distinguished from Groups II and III only for the 2nd-, 3rd-, and 4th-degree relatives.

Table 2 indicates that for 32 of the 52 probands (62%) of Group I there were other twin sets in addition to the first set, which defined a positive family history. An "excess" of twins was determined to be those twins beyond the first two sets. This is considered a strongly positive family history. A total of 74 excess twin sets was noted for these 32 families, indicating an average of 2.3 excess twins for each such family, or an average of 3.3 nonproband twins for each. The combined data from Tables 1–3 indicate that when starting from twin probands, about 74% (52/70) have a positive family history and that 62% of the latter (32/52) or 44% of the total (32/70) have a strongly positive family history (ie at least three twin sets), and therefore at least a portion of twins may be forecast by a strongly positive family history. Similar figures were obtained when families with only DZ twin pairs were excluded, indicating that MZ twins also reflect heritable influences.

Out of the 70 families in Group I, there were 52 instances (74%) in which at least one additional twin set was present as genetic relatives to the proband twin

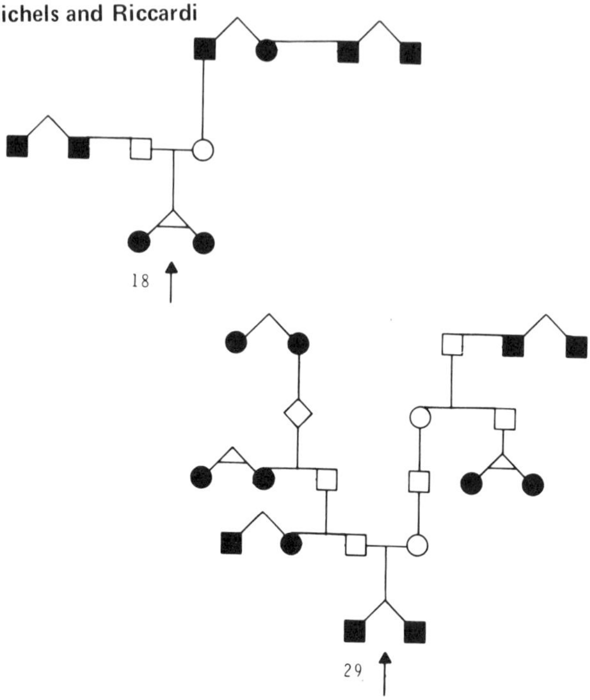

Fig. 3. Representative pedigrees suggesting heritability of twinning through both males and females. Note discordance of zygosity.

set (Table 2). The degree of relatedness between the proband twins and the closest twin set was noted for each family (Table 3): 7% as first-degree relatives, 24% as second-degree, 20% as third-degree, and 23% as fourth-degree. These percentages, plus acknowledgment of specific pedigrees (Figs. 2–5), have indicated to us an important heritable component to twinning in at least some instances. Heritability is emphasized when these percentages are compared to similar data for Groups II and III (Table 3), although there is an awareness bias for twins in Group I; and in Groups II and III inadequate histories probably result in a factitiously small number of twins in the second-, third-, and fourth-degree categories.

Figure 6 exemplifies the awareness bias that is probably intrinsic to Group I parents: an inordinate awareness of twinning among family members. The closest related twin set to the proband set is a sixth-degree relative.

DISCUSSION

The heritability of twinning is often considered to be restricted to dizygosity and to influences through the maternal line. Large retrospective twin studies by

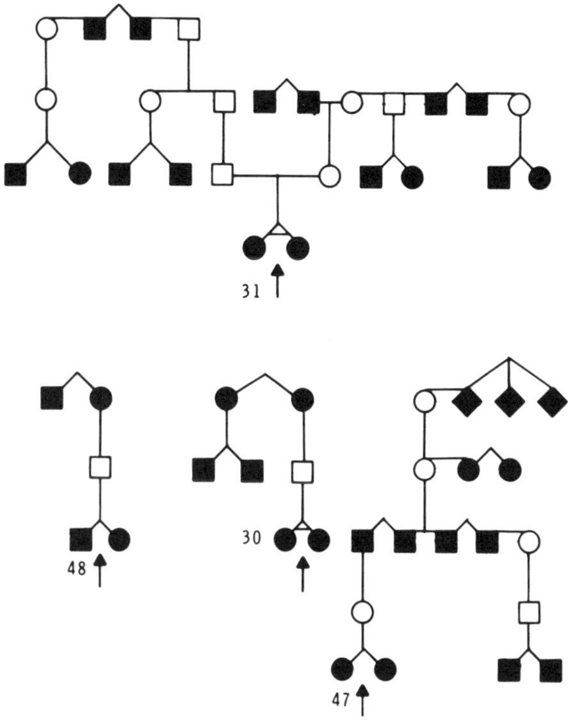

Fig. 4. Representative pedigrees showing clustering of twins within families; up to 5 sets in family 47.

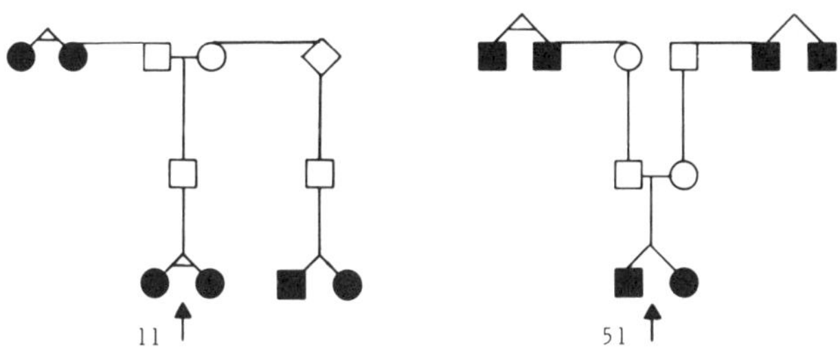

Fig. 5. Representative pedigrees. See text and Figure 2 legend. Note both MZ and DZ twins.

Weinberg [6] and later Bulmer [4] showed that the repeat frequency of twinning (ie the frequency of twinning among women who already had one set of twins) was increased only for dizygotic twins. However, assessments of recurrence only among sibs may be too restrictive. Our data show that when starting

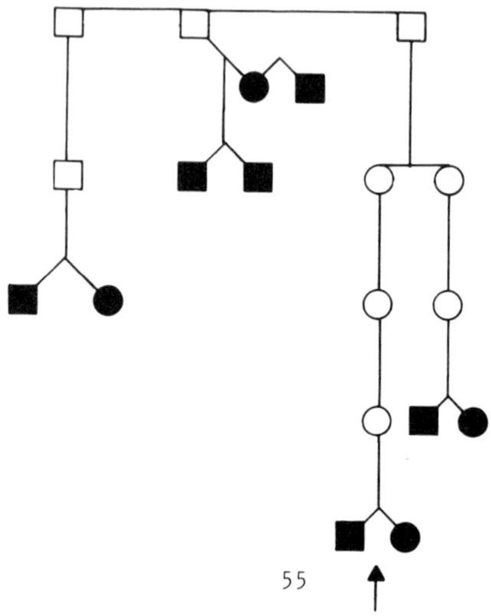

Fig. 6. Sample pedigree exemplifying awareness bias in Group I: Set of twins closest to proband set is 6th-degree relative.

from proband twins, 74% of families (52/70) will have a positive family history for one or more additional twin sets, and of these, 62% (32/52) will include at least three twin sets related as first-, second-, third-, and/or fourth-degree relatives (Tables 1 and 2). When this is compared to the lesser likelihood of finding similar frequencies of families with twin clustering if the proband was not ascertained because he/she is a twin (Groups II and III), the presence of a positive family history for two or more nonproband twin sets indicates an increased risk for twinning (Tables 3 and 4). Moreover, in these high-risk families both MZ and DZ twins may be involved (Table 1) and the risk applies to the offspring of male as well as female relatives (Figs. 1–5). A heritable aspect of monozygosity would not necessarily be reflected in prior studies of repeat frequency of twinning [4], since only first-degree relatives were considered. In contrast, since our primary study population (Group I) was biased for more than one set of twins per family over several generations, we therefore may have selected families in which twinning is heritable.

Weinberg [6] found an increased twinning rate among first-degree relatives of mothers of twins but not among the fathers. In 63% (20/32) of families in Group I who had three or more sets of twins related as first- to fourth-degree relatives, a male intermediary was present and would have had to transmit any

TABLE 4. Proportions (%) of Families With Excess Twin Sets as a Function of Relatedness of Two Closest Sets*

	1°	2°	3°	4°	Other
Group I	1.5	17.1	11.4	15.7	1.5
Group II	0	1.7	0	0	1.7
Group III	7.1	1.5	0	0	0

*Excess twins are noted for only the 2nd-, 3rd-, and 4th-degree subgroups of Group I suggesting that multiple generations need to be considered to appreciate familial twin clustering.

heritable factor. This large percentage makes it unlikely that these instances were coincidental. A twinning diathesis heritable through the paternal line may not be evident in a study in which large pedigrees are not looked at, since appreciation of multiple-generation involvement may be important. Studies of families ascertained through twin organizations may select for these families with twins in multiple generations and show that in some families male inheritance is an important factor. Our data are corroborated by a recent report by Harvey et al [5] of several families in which genetic factors seem to play a role in determining MZ twinning with apparent transmission of MZ twinning through males or females.

The incidence of families in which the proband or the index case has a twin set as first-degree relatives is approximately the same for Groups I, II, and III. Therefore, a positive family history among first-degree relatives alone had little value in predicting recurrence. We then calculated the percentage of families in Group I in which there were more than two sets of twins as a function of their degree of relatedness (Table 4). The proportions were 1.5% for first-degree, 17.1% for second-degree, 11.4% for third-degree, and 15.7% for fourth-degree. These numbers are consistent with a relatively high risk for familial twinning in the second-, third-, and fourth-degree subgroups. The reason this phenomenon is not reflected in the subgroup with first-degree relatives as twins is not clear. Thus the data from Tables 2–4 show that there are certain families with strong clustering of twins, up to five sets per family. We interpret this to mean that a history of two or more twin sets in the family of a couple presenting for amniocentesis, constitutes a reasonable basis for performing ultrasound.

Group III served as a control in that the original proband presented for genetic counseling for reasons other than twinning. These 70 families allowed us to assess how frequently genetically related twin sets would be apparent when primary ascertainment (ie clinic referral) was irrespective of twins and the pedigrees were taken by various examiners with no particular attention paid to twinning. The percentage of families with a negative family history for twins beyond the index case was the same as in Group II (76%) and distinct from Group I (Table 3).

The fact that the number of twin second-, third-, and fourth-degree relatives in Groups II and III was less than in Group I led us to believe that families in Group I were more aware of twins (exemplified in Fig. 6). Detection of no fourth-degree relatives in Group III lent support to this. This type of bias presumably contributes to some of Group I's positive family histories, especially in some of those families with an excess of twins (ie more than two sets). Although this type of bias makes comparison between the three study groups more difficult, and suggests that more careful family histories may be necessary before twin recurrence is deemed unlikely, we do not feel that this bias alone explains our strongly positive family histories (as defined above). The number of twins seen in each of these families is more than one would expect given average family sizes and a twinning rate of 1/80 [7].

CONCLUSION

We reasoned that if we started out with families biased for multiple twin sets over several generations, we might be able to discern legitimate heritability factors not apparent in larger surveys restricted to recurrence of twins only among first-degree relatives. Our major limitation, however, was to ensure that the original bias did not factitiously account for apparent genetic influences. We feel that our families with three or more twin sets, in the context of expected numbers of twins and comparisons with the two control groups, do indeed demonstrate a genetically based twin recurrence risk for some families, and that both MZ and DZ twinning and male-mediated influences are contributory. We thus suggest that a positive family history for two or more sets of twins related as first- to fourth-degree relatives to the pregnancy through either the mother or father is a reasonable basis for selecting couples at risk for twinning, thereby justifying the additional cost and effort involved in preamniocentesis ultrasound if it is not done routinely.

EDITORIAL COMMENTS

This paper calls attention to the idea that an investigation of first-degree relatives of twin pairs is not adequate in assessing heritability of twinning, that heritability factors play a role in monozygotic as well as dizygotic twinning, that similar factors might predispose both to monozygotic and dizygotic twinning and that heritability might involve the paternal as well as the maternal line.

The reader should *not* be mislead to the conclusion that only in families containing two or more sets of twins is preamniocentesis ultrasonography indicated. In the editor's opinion, ultrasonography should precede *any* amniocentesis performed for genetic reasons in midtrimester. While reasons in addition to the detection of twins (such as placental localization, assessment of fetal viability, pregnancy staging, and a search for grossly discernible malformations) make preamniocentesis ultrasonography mandatory, a critical assessment for the presence of multiple pregnancy should be an integral part of *any* preamniocentesis ultrasonogram.

Robert L. Summitt

ACKNOWLEDGMENTS

Thanks to Ms. G. Giesige, the Milwaukee Mothers of Twins Club and the Organizaion of Twin-Blessed Mothers for cooperating in the data collection. Thanks also to Ms. C. Gibson for assistance in manuscript preparation.

REFERENCES

1. Milunsky A: Current concepts in genetics: Prenatal diagnosis of genetic disorders. N Engl J Med 295:377, 1976.
2. Grennert L, Persson PH, Gennser GZ, Kullander S: Ultrasound and human placental lactogen screening for early detection of twin pregnancies. Lancet 1:4, 1976.
3. The NICHD National Registry for Amniocentesis Study Group: Midtrimester amniocentesis for prenatal diagnosis. JAMA 236:1471, 1976.
4. Bulmer MG: "The Biology of Twinning in Man." Oxford: Clarendon Press, 1970.
5. Harvey MAS, Huntley RMC, Smith DW: Familial monozygotic twinning. J Pediatr 90: 246, 1977.
6. Weinberg W: Die Anlage zur Mehrlingsgeburt beim Menschen und ihre Vererbung. Arch Rass-u Ges Biol 6:322–339, 470–482, 609–630, 1909. (Cited in Bulmer MG. op cit.)
7. Benirschke K, Chung KK: Multiple pregnancy. N Engl J Med 288:1276, 1973.

Dicephalus Dipus Tribrachius Conjoined Twins in a Female Infant*

Andrew Hamon, MD and Nuhad Dinno, MD

The birth of conjoined twins is a rare phenomenon. Robertson [1] and Hanson [2] assess the incidence of conjoined twins at approximately 1/50,000 births. Symmetric conjoined twins are rare, and asymmetric twins are even less common.

Buchta reports an incidence of anencephaly at 1/1,000 births [3]. If the two anomalies are unrelated, then the combination of these two defects is extremely rare.

It is the purpose of this paper to report an unusual case of dicephalus dipus tribrachius with one anencephalic head. An extensive search of the literature showed no similar case report.

CASE HISTORY

This unusual conjoined twin was born to nonconsanguineous parents. During pregnancy the Rh-negative mother was monitored for Rh-antibody titers, which did not exceed 1:8. The mother had a prior history of syphilis, but the VDRL test was negative during this pregnancy.

At 36 weeks of gestation, during a routine office visit, the physician noted fetal decelerations. An oxytocin challenge test was positive. Amniocentesis returned thick, dark green, meconium-stained fluid, and a cesarean section was performed. Conjoined twins were delivered through a low transverse cervical incision. The initial Apgar score was 1, and the twins died within 30 minutes.

The placenta was monochorionic and monoamniotic, with a velamentous attached umbilical cord. Three vessels were present.

*From the Department of Obstetrics and Gynecology, Department of Pediatrics, University of Louisville, School of Medicine, Louisville, Kentucky.

Birth Defects: Original Article Series, Volume XIV, Number 6A, pages 213–218

These black twins (Fig. 1) weighed 2,420 gm and had a crown–rump length of 39 cm. The left twin was anencephalic and had a large occipital meningo-encephalocele. The right twin had a normal head, with a cleft lip the only anomaly. The twins were conjoined from the shoulder to the sacrum. They had two normal-appearing lateral arms and an abnormal median arm. The external genitalia were those of a female infant. There were two lower limbs.

FAMILY HISTORY

The father is 25 years of age and has a sister who gave birth to twin sons. The mother is 19 years of age. Her mother also gave birth to conjoined twins who died shortly after birth (Fig. 2), and apparently one of those also had anencephaly. Two arms and four legs were present. Several sets of normal twins were reported on the mother's side of the family, as shown by the pedigree (Fig. 2). The parents are unrelated.

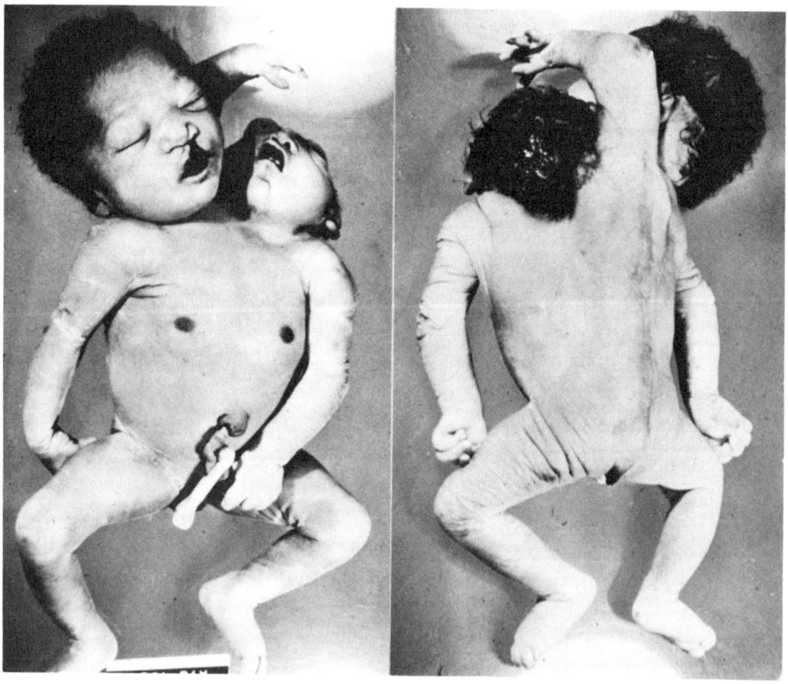

Fig 1. Front and back view of conjoined twins.

RADIOLOGIC EVALUATION

Radiologic evaluation revealed soft tissue fusion from the shoulder to the pelvis, with duplication of the entire spinal column joined at a single pelvis (Fig. 3). The bony thorax was separate laterally and shared, by a fusion of the ribs, in the midline. A common median forearm contained three long bones, one ulna and two radii (Fig. 4).

AUTOPSY

Additional findings revealed the respiratory system to be entirely duplicated with four hypoplastic lungs. There was a single pericardial sac with two hearts joined at a common midline atrium. The aortas and their branches were duplicated. The aortas joined at the 4th lumbar vertebra for a distance of 1 cm, then divided, and one vessel entered each leg. The venae cavae were normal. The mirror-image chambers and valves of the heart were normal except for the common atrium.

The thymus, thyroid, parathyroid glands, and pancreas were duplicated. The liver was large, fused at the midline and had two gallbladders, one in the midline and one at the right lateral margin (Fig. 5). There was a single normal spleen.

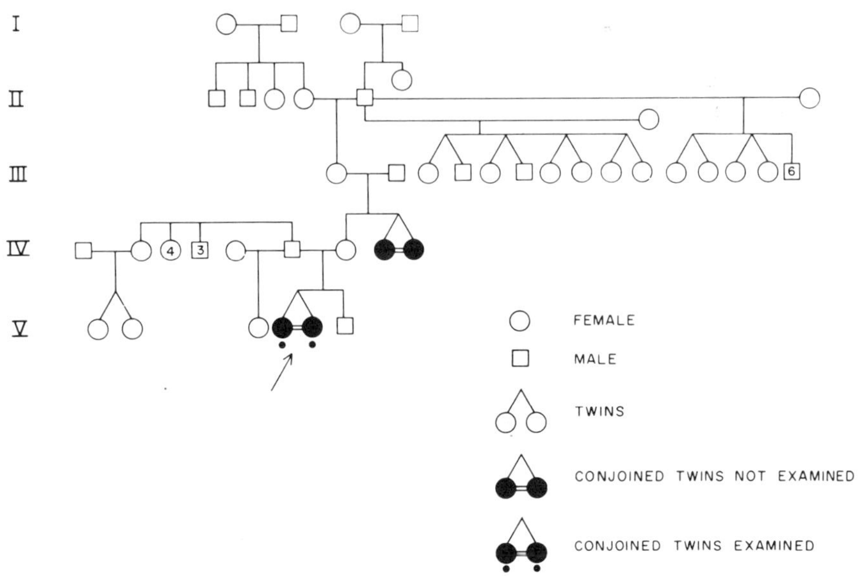

Fig. 2. Pedigree analysis showing high incidence of twinning on maternal side.

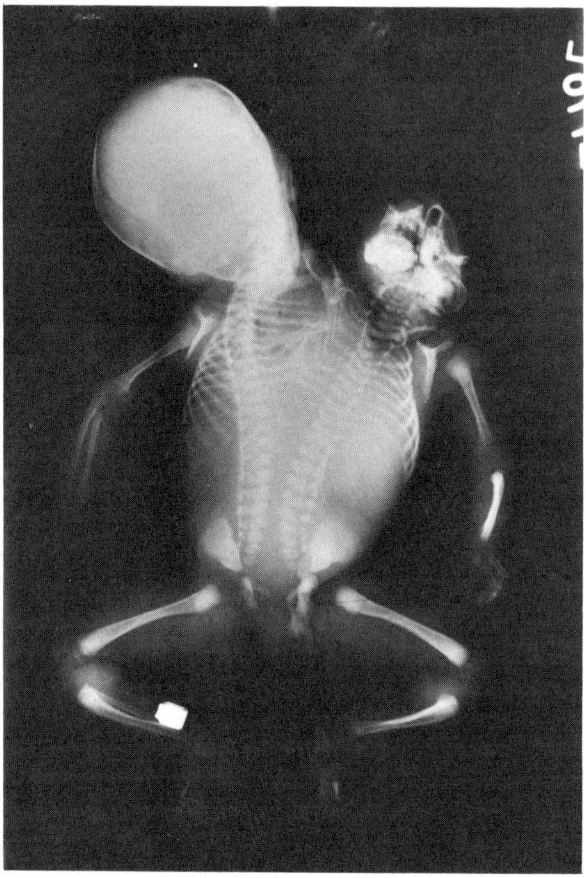

Fig. 3. Radiogram of the conjoined twins.

The alimentary system was duplicated from the mouth to the distal ilium. The remainder of the system was single and apparently normal.

The urogenital system was single and normal, and two adrenal glands were present in the normal location. However, two fused adrenal glands were also present in the midline just below the diaphragm.

Microscopic evaluation of the tissues revealed necrosis of the brain. There was primary atelectasis of the lungs with acute congestion and foci of inspissated amniotic fluid. The spleen and liver were acutely congested. The colon was aganglionic. No diagnostic abnormalities of the heart, upper gastrointestinal tract, adrenals, thymus, thyroid gland, pancreas, or umbilical cord could be found.

Chromosome analysis of blood by G banding, with fibroblast cultures from both heads, revealed a normal female karyotype.

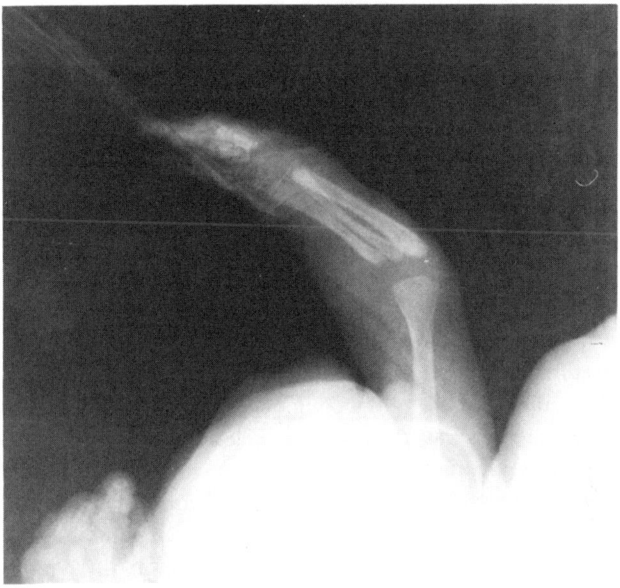

Fig. 4. Abnormal median arm roentgenogram showing two radii and one ulna.

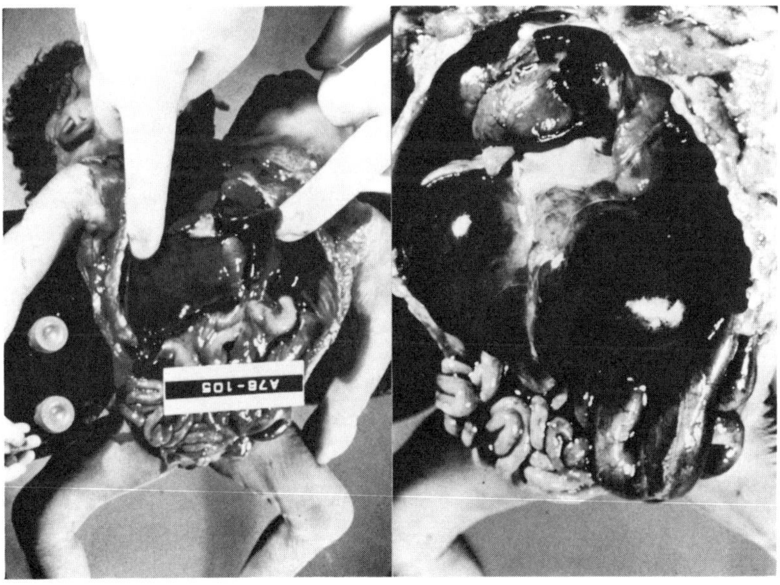

Fig. 5. Two views of the viscera and thoracic cage.

DISCUSSION

It is generally believed that conjoined twins are derived from a single blastocyst and represent a form of monozygotic twinning. They are united because the embryonic cells fail to separate completely in the process of division [4]. These twins are of the same sex, which supports the theory of monozygotic derivation. It is generally agreed that the cause of conjoined twinning is unknown but that the variations in the types of twins are related to the time during gestation of interference with the division of the inner cell mass [5]. The spectrum of possibilities in such cases may range from parasitic monsters or conjoined twins to two monozygotic twins.

Our case represents one of the more unusual types of conjoined twins, with some findings similar to those in the conjoined twins discussed by Potter [6]. The twins in our case were asymmetric with one twin having typical anencephaly. The monochorionic, monoamniotic placenta with a single umbilical cord further supports the concept of aberrant monozygotic twins. Similar normal fibroblast cultures obtained from each head rule out a chromosomal etiology.

Of special interest in this instance is the fact that a sib of the mother was a conjoined stillbirth, also with apparent anencephaly. This will be important in any future pregnancies, since the prospect for subsequent twin malformation is 25 times greater in this mother than in the general population [7]. The prognosis for development of a neural tube defect is even greater [8]. The knowledge that this mother is at high risk will warrant close observation during future pregnancies with amniocentesis and other diagnostic tests by which a fetal abnormality might be detected.

REFERENCES

1. Robertson EG: Craniopagus parietalis. Arch Neurol Psychiatr 70:189, 1953.
2. Hanson JW: Incidence of conjoined twinning. Lancet 2:1257, 1975.
3. Buchta RM: Anencephaly in female thoracopagus conjoined twins. Clin Pediatr 12:598, 1973.
4. Guttmacher AF, Nichols BL: Teratology of conjoined twins. In Bergsma D (ed): "Conjoined Twins." White Plains: The National Foundation–March of Dimes, BD:OAS III(1): 3–9, 1967.
5. Zimmermann AA: Embryologic and anatomic considerations of conjoined twins. In "Conjoined Twins," ibid pp 18–27.
6. Potter EL, Criag JM: "Pathology of the Fetus and the Infant." Chicago: Year Book Medical Publishers, 1975, pp 220–237.
7. Rudolph AJ, Michaels JP, Nichols BL: Obstetric management of conjoined twins. In "Conjoined Twins," op cit pp 28–37.
8. Warkany J: "Congenital Malformations, Notes & Comments." Chicago: Year Book Medical Publishers, 1971, pp 189–200.

Genetic Etiology for Monozygotic Twinning*

Lawrence R. Shapiro, MD, Lionel Zemek, MD, and
Martin J. Shulman, MD

Genetic factors in the etiology of dizygotic twins are known to exist, whereas no genetic factors have been thought to be related to monozygotic twinning. Except for a few instances [1, 2] the literature on twins has dismissed familial instances of monozygotic twinning as chance occurrences or due to ascertainment bias [3]. A recent report by Harvey et al [2] has presented ten families with multiple instances of monozygotic twins. In their report, zygosity was determined clinically and with blood type analysis in only two of the families. Pedigree analysis of these ten families suggested a single gene dominant mode of transmission with variable penetrance and vertical transmission from male to female.

The purpose of this paper is to present a single extended family with four sets of monozygotic twins (Fig. 1). The family consists of a pair of monozygotic female twins, of whom one has had two sets of monozygotic male twins and the other has had three male singletons. A female maternal cousin, once removed, of the female twins has had one set of female monozygotic twins and one male singleton. There are no associated diseases of morphologic abnormalities.

Zygosity determinations included clinical examination, dermatoglyphic analysis, and quantitative blood typing of erythrocytes in all of the twins. Physical examination, as illustrated by the photographs of each set of twins, confirmed their identical appearance. Great difficulty in distinguishing one twin from another was encountered despite the fact that they were dressed differently. In addition, eye and hair color was identical within each twin set. Dermatoglyphic analysis according to the method of Holt [4] revealed the highest possible probability for monozygosity in each twin set. Quantitative blood typing of erythrocytes in all twins was done by the method of Berkman et al [5], which is

*This work was supported in part by the New York State Department of Health Birth Defects Institute and The National Foundation–March of Dimes.

Birth Defects: Original Article Series, Volume XIV, Number 6A, pages 219–222

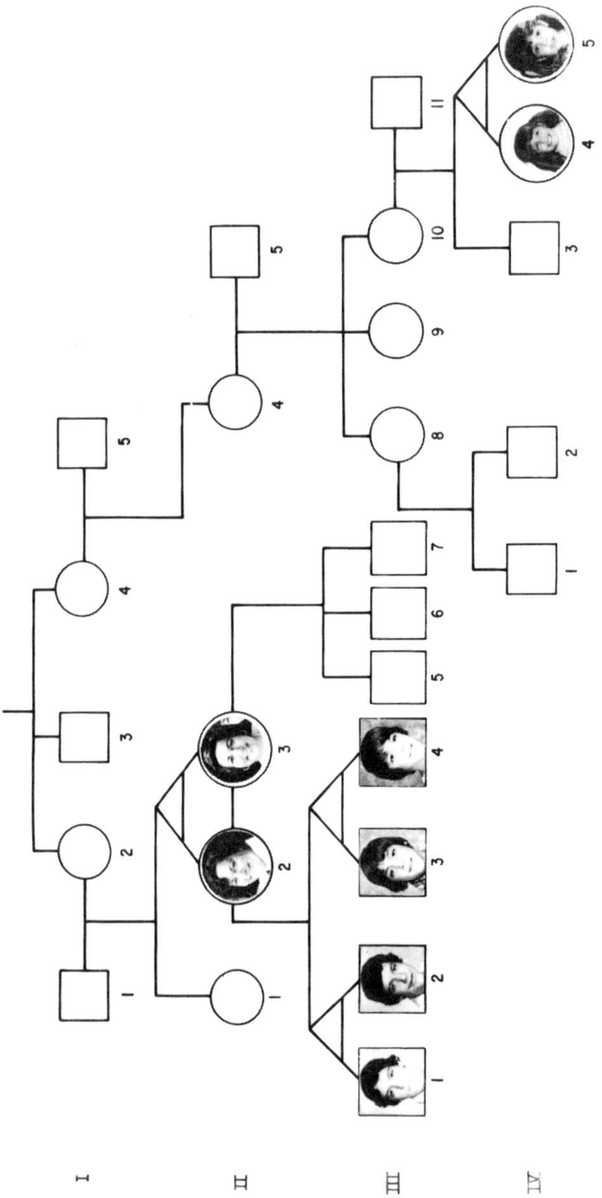

Fig. 1. Pedigree of single extended family with four sets of monozygotic twins.

an automated and sequential quantitation of blood typing profiles of human erythrocytes. This method has been found to be extremely accurate and does not require analysis of the parents for comparison purposes, although this was done for three of the four twin pairs. The quantitative blood typing profiles of each of the twins confirmed that they all were monozygotic (Fig. 2).

The four pairs of twins of the families presented above and those previously reported tend to support a single gene autosomal dominant mode of inheritance with variable penetrance for some cases of monozygotic twinning. In the absence of observed male-to-female vertical transmission in this small sample, no conclusions can be drawn regarding maternal or paternal effects. Previous studies have indicated that familial instances of repeated monozygotic twinning are relatively uncommon especially when compared to the incidence of familial dizygotic twinning [6].

Monozygotic twinning can be considered to be an early alteration in morphogenesis, and the increased incidence of chromosome abnormalities in monozygotic twins [7] provides indirect support of this view. When one does consider monozygotic twinning as an early alteration of morphogenesis, it is not surprising that some of the modes of developmental pathology may be related to genetic factors and that an autosomal dominant mode of inheritance for some forms of monozygotic twins does exist, albeit uncommonly.

ACKNOWLEDGMENTS

The authors wish to express their gratitude to Richard E. Rosenfield, MD, Director of the Department of Blood Bank and Clinical Microscopy, The Mount

Δ Log O.D. x 10^2

	Rh									Kell					Mn				JK		Fy		Le		ABO
	1	2	3	4	5	6	7	8	10	1	2	3	4	6	M	N	S	s	a	b	a	b	a	b	
II·2	44	/	/	15	46	24	20	/	/	/	38	16	21	/	41	/	44	+	36	/	36	/			A
II·3	57	/	/	22	65	15	28	/	/	/	50	24	26	/	27	/	30	+	48	/	22	/			A
III·1	64	/	/	33	69	40	30	/	/	/	45	/	13	/	49	/	51	+	/	/	/	/			A
III·2	59	/	/	28	67	25	33	/	/	/	38	/	9	/	52	13	48	+	/	/	/	/			A
III·3	57	/	/	30	34	30	23	/	/	/	49	27	30	/	37	/	56	/	46	/	/	/			A
III·4	61	/	/	30	70*	16	32	/	/	/	55	27	30	/	25	/	61	/	32	/	/	/			A
IV·4	21	/	/	90	46	31	/	/	/	/	41	/	22	/	/	+	+	+	44	/	/	/		41	A
IV·5	17	/	/	87	48	39	/	/	/	/	41	/	20	/		+	+	+	48	/	/	/		48	A

Fig. 2. Quantitative blood typing profiles of each of the twins. The asterisk indicates a technical error.

Sinai Hospital, New York City, for performing the quantitative blood typing profiles of each of the twins.

REFERENCES

1. Gedda L, Russo O, Capone M: Heredity of twinning in families of MZ twins. Acta Genet Med Gemellol (Roma) 23:18, 1974 (Special issue).
2. Harvey MAS, Huntley RMC, Smith DW: Familial monozygotic twinning. J Pediatr 90:246–248, 1977.
3. Stern O: "Principles of Human Genetics." 2nd Ed. San Francisco: W. H. Freeman, 1960, p 541.
4. Holt SB: "The Genetics of Dermal Ridges." Springfield: Charles C Thomas, 1968, pp 80–81.
5. Berkman EM, Nusbacher J, Kochwa S, Rosenfield RE: Quantitative blood typing profiles of human erythrocytes. Transfusion 11:317–332, 1971.
6. Myrianthopoulos WC: An epidemiologic survey of twins in a large prospectively studied population. Am J Hum Genet 22:611–629, 1970.
7. Nance WE, Uchida I: Turner's syndrome, twinning and an unusual variant of glucose-6-phosphate dehydrogenase. Am J Hum Genet 16:380–392, 1964.

Discordance in Monozygotic Twins for Aglossia-Adactylia, and Possible Clues to the Pathogenesis of the Syndrome

Meinhard Robinow, MD, J.L. Marsh, MD, Milton T. Edgerton, MD, Hernan Sabio, MD, and G. F. Johnson, MD

Certain congenital malformation syndromes with overlapping manifestations constitute a "family" of syndromes. Gorlin et al [1] call this group the "Oromandibular-limb hypogenesis syndromes"; Grosse and Wiedemann [2] use the term "Oroacral malformations." These syndromes include aglossia-adactylia, syndactyly-ankyloglossia, glossopalatine ankylosis, Hanhart syndrome, and Charlie M. syndrome. The spectrum of manifestations includes the following dysmorphic features:

Face	Bilateral 6th and 7th nerve paralysis (Möbius syndrome) Cleft lip and/or cleft palate
Tongue	Aglossia, microglossia, ankyloglossia
Oral cavity	Intraoral bands
Teeth	Partial anodontia
Mandible	Hypoplasia, collapse of dental arch
Limbs	Reduction deformities (amputations, oligodactyly, symbrachydactyly)

The "aglossia" varies from moderate reduction to virtual absence. Similarly, the limb defects may range from loss of a single digit to amputation of an entire limb (Fig. 1). (In this context, the term "amputation" is used to designate loss or absence of a distal limb part, regardless of the mechanism producing it.)

Birth Defects: Original Article Series, Volume XIV, Number 6A, pages 223–230

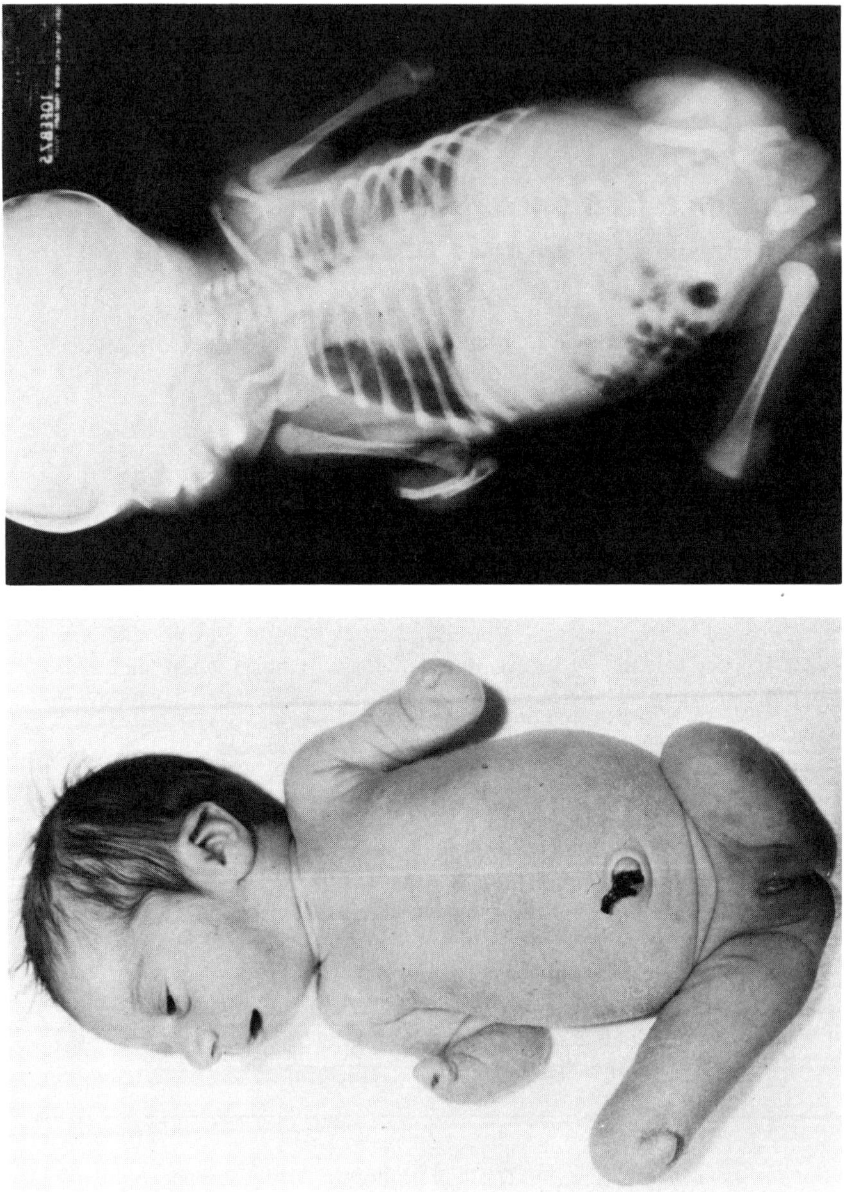

Fig. 1. Unusually severe limb defects in a 4-day-old infant girl with aglossia-adactylia. Note also the severe micrognathia.

The cause and pathogenesis of the syndromes have been obscure. Genetic factors seem unlikely. Chromosome studies have always been normal [3]. No familial cases have been reported, though Temtamy and McKusick found clefts and dental anomalies in some of their patients' relatives [4]. Finally, the limb defects are always asymmetric, an uncommon finding in genetic disorders. We have selected from a larger group three cases with features that may shed some light on the pathogenesis of these syndromes.

CASE REPORTS

Case 1 was one of twin boys whose parents were second cousins (Fig. 2). The mother had experienced cramping and intermittent bleeding throughout the pregnancy. At birth the patient weighed 2.4 kg. His co-twin weighed 3.3 kg. There was a single placenta. Immunogenetic studies proved the twins to be monozygotic (Table 1). The close resemblance of their hair, eyes, ears, and noses contrasts with the greatly differing mid- and lower facial features (Fig. 3).

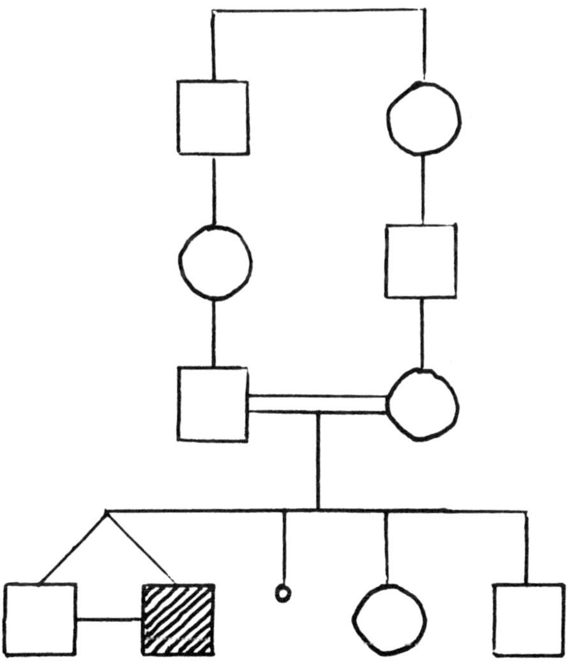

Fig. 2. *Case 1*, pedigree.

TABLE 1. Probability That Twins (*Case 1*) Are Monozygotic*

	F	M	□ ^	□	P dizygosity
Sex	M	F	M	M	1/2
MN	MM	MN	MM	MM	1/2
Le′	+	0	0	0	1/2
Le″	0	+	+	+	1/2
Duffy (Fy^a)	+	0	0	0	1/2
Stoltzfuss	+	0	0	0	1/2
Adenosine deaminase	1/1	2/1	2/1	2/1	1/2
Alkaline phosphatase	D/C	A/B	B/B	B/B	1/4
Group-specific proteins	1/1	2/1	1/1	1/1	1/2

Combined P dizygosity	$0.7 \times (1/2)^{10} = 0.0007$
P monozygosity	$1.0 - 0.0007 = 0.9993$

*The rows list sex, erythrocyte antigens, and serum proteins for which the parents (F,M) are discordant and the twins (□ ^ □) are concordant. The last column gives the probabilities that dizygotic twins are concordant for the listed traits. The combined P dizygosity is the relative probability of dizygotic twinning multiplied by the product of the individual P dizygosity.

The patient had the following features of the syndrome: 6th and 7th nerve paralysis (Möbius syndrome), ankyloglossia and severe hypoglossia, micrognathia and retrognathia, syndactyly of all fingers, right hand (Fig. 4a), oligo- and microdactyly, left hand (Fig. 4a), amputation, left foot (Fig. 4b), and right clubfoot.

Now, at the age of 6 years, after many corrective procedures, his eyes are straight, the syndactylous fingers are separated, and the tongue tip is free. His speech is marked by a minor articulation defect. He is achieving well in school. His twin brother is 8 cm taller and is completely unaffected.

The presence of the syndrome in only one of monozygotic twins suggests that some nongenetic intrauterine factor is involved in the pathogenesis.

Case 2 provided a clue to the teratogenic mechanism. The patient was a one-day-old infant girl with microglossia and amputation of several fingers and toes. She had failed to pass meconium and had developed abdominal distention. Intestinal obstruction was diagnosed. At surgery she presented the findings of the "apple peel bowel" [5]. This anomaly consists of atresia of the distal duodenum and proximal jejunum. Beyond the obstruction the caliber of the bowel is reduced and its posterior mesentery is absent. The term "apple peel" describes the characteristic coiling of the miniaturized small intestine. A constant finding in

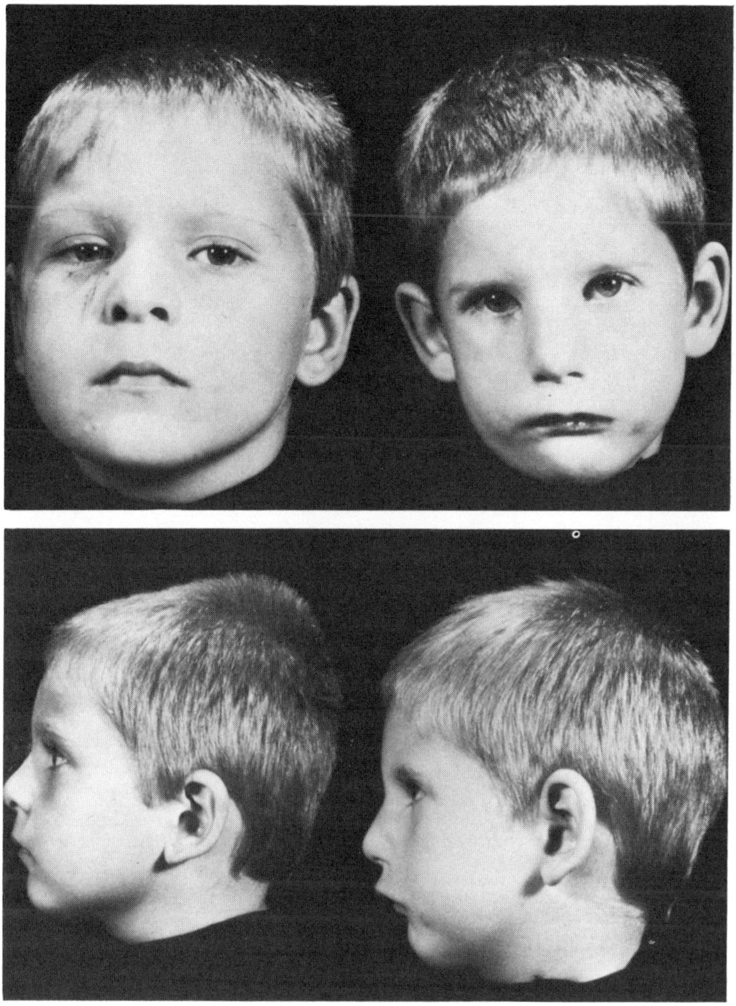

Fig. 3. *Case 1.* The affected member of the monozygotic pair (right) has 7th nerve paralysis and micrognathia.

the apple peel bowel and its presumptive cause is obliteration of the superior mesenteric artery (Fig. 5).

Case 3. The third patient in this series had an asymmetric microglossia (more severe reduction on the right), micrognathia, and multiple limb amputations. In addition, he had a single kidney, another anomaly that conceivably could have been caused by an intrauterine vascular occlusion.

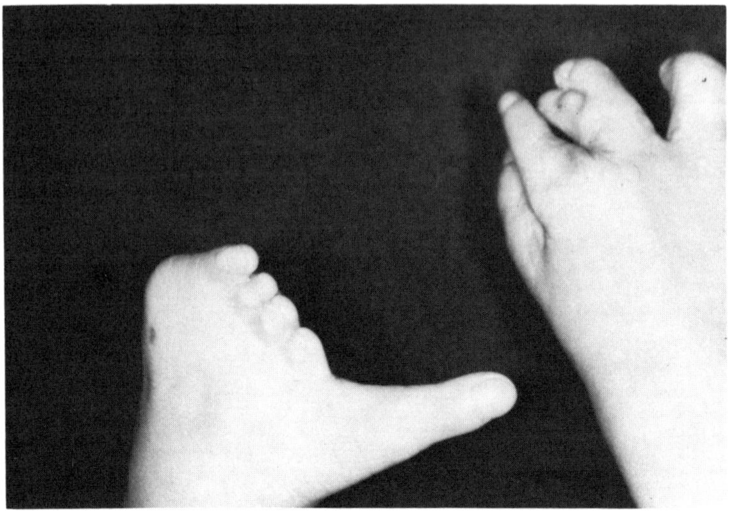

Fig. 4a. Syndactyly, right hand (after surgery); oligomicrodactyly, left hand.

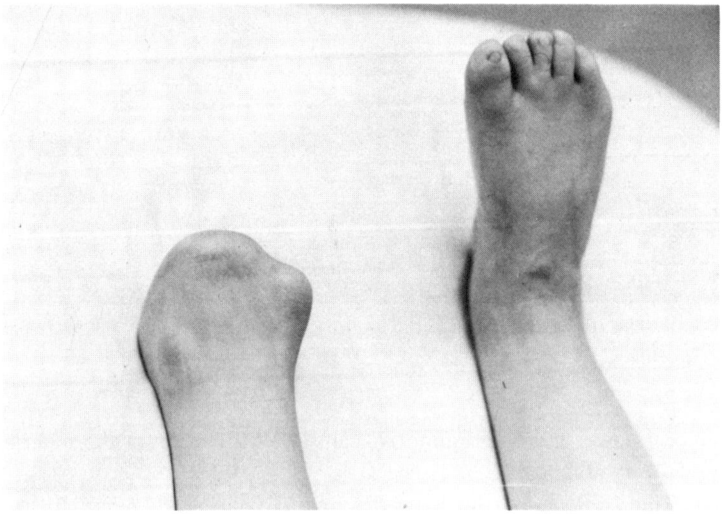

Fig. 4b.Amputation left foot.

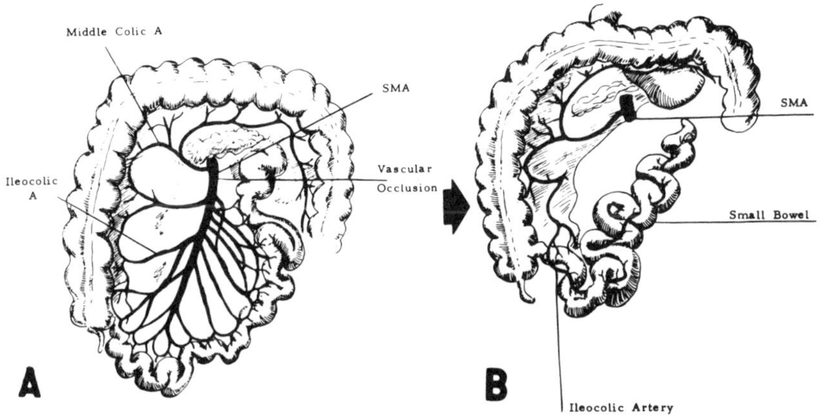

Fig. 5. Apple peel bowel. Reproduced from Leonidas et al [5] with permission.

DISCUSSION

Animal models have been developed that lend further support to the vascular hypothesis. Jost [6, 7] has produced congenital deformities of the jaws and limbs by injection of adrenalin and pitressin into fetal rats and rabbits as well as by dehydration of the dams. The fetal lesions consisted of edema, followed by hemorrhage and necrosis. Very similar hemorrhagic lesions were found to occur spontaneously in the paws of genetically brachydactylous mice and rabbits. The lesions could be produced only during a relatively brief critical period of fetal development.

D.E. Poswillo has observed "lesions of the periphery, particularly hypodactylia and occasionally fusion of the lips and anomalies of the lower jaw" and commented that "these lesions appear to be closely related to hemorrhage, which we can induce by pressor agents injected into the peritoneal cavity of the dam" [personal communication]. If timing of these defects in man is limited, as in rats and rabbits, the most likely period of risk would be between 6 and 8 weeks of fetal development. At that time the limbs have divided into upper, middle, and distal parts; the digits may or may not yet be separated; and lip and palate are closing.

In conclusion, we propose that some vascular accident, followed by tissue necrosis, is an important step in the pathogenesis of the aglossia-adactylia syndrome. Conceivably, such an event is in some cases facilitated by a genetic predisposition.

ACKNOWLEDGMENTS

The contributions of Mrs. S. Krovaad, Blood Bank, University of Virginia Hospital, and of Mrs. N.L. Delaney, Johns Hopkins Immunogenetic Laboratory, to the immunogenetic studies reported in *Case 1* are gratefully acknowledged.

REFERENCES

1. Gorlin RJ, Pindborg JJ, Cohen MM: "Syndromes of the Head and Neck." 2nd Ed. New York: McGraw-Hill, 1976.
2. Grosse FR, Wiedemann H: Syndromes with reduction and surplus anomalies of the hand. In Bergsma D, Lenz W (eds): "Morphogenesis and Malformation of the Limb." New York: Alan R. Liss for The National Foundation–March of Dimes. BD:OAS XIII(1): 301–318, 1977.
3. Nevin NC, Burrows D, Allen D, Kernohan DC: Aglossia-adactylia syndrome. J Med Genet 12:89–93, 1975.
4. Temtamy S, McKusick VA: Synopsis of hand malformations with particular emphasis on genetic factors. In Bergsma D (ed): Part III "Limb Malformations." New York: The National Foundation–March of Dimes. BD:OAS V(3):125–184, 1969.
5. Leonidas JC et al: Duodenal atresia with "apple peel" small bowel. Radiology 118:661–665, 1976.
6. Jost A: La dégénérescence des extrémités de rat sous les actions hormonales (acroblepsie expérimentale) et la théorie des bulles myélencéphaliques de Bonnevie. Arch Fr Pediatr 10:1–6, 1953.
7. Jost A, Roof J, Courtat M: Congenital amputations determined by the BR gene and those induced by adrenalin injection in the rabbit fetus. In "Limb Development and Deformity: Problems of Evaluation and Rehabilitation." Springfield: Charles C Thomas, 1969.

Index